# The Training of Good Physicians

# THE TRAINING OF GOOD PHYSICIANS

**Critical Factors in Career Choices**

by Fremont J. Lyden / H. Jack Geiger / Osler L. Peterson

A COMMONWEALTH FUND BOOK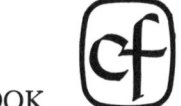

Harvard University Press, Cambridge, Massachusetts / 1968

© Copyright 1968 by the President and Fellows of Harvard College
All rights reserved

Distributed in Great Britain by Oxford University Press, London

Library of Congress Catalog Card Number 68–21977

Printed in the United States of America

# Acknowledgments

A RETROSPECTIVE STUDY of the training and career decisions of nearly two thousand physicians who graduated from twelve widely scattered medical schools required unusual care in planning. We were particularly fortunate to have the frequent advice and help of Dr. Sol Levine during the preparatory phase of the study reported here. His help was both detailed (as in the construction of the questionnaire) and of a more general character, as when we outlined the steps to be taken to assure a high response rate. Edwin B. Hutchins of the Association of American Medical Colleges assisted us greatly in selecting medical schools for inclusion in this study and also made available the Medical College Admission Test Scores for the physicians in our study population.

The extensive statistical work that was necessary to produce the several hundred tables upon which our results are based was organized and completed by Mrs. Mary Wood McDonald. Her meticulous attention to detail and her competent and systematic completion of tables was a vital first step in data handling. Miss Katharine Hendrie, who performed a large number of statistical computations, programmed much of our material for computer treatment, and patiently checked our many tables and figures to assure their accuracy, has been of inestimable help in completing this volume.

A special note of thanks is due to the deans and assistant deans of twelve medical schools who aided us by supplying information about the medical school records of their graduates and whose assistance in follow-up of nonresponders contributed very importantly to the overall results and especially to the very high response rate achieved. Our preoccupation with obtaining a very high response rate led us, possibly unnecessarily, to assure each school that the fact of its participation would be held in confidence. This makes it impossible for us to identify individually the many medical school officers whose help has been so great.

This study could not have been done without the cooperation of nearly two thousand practicing doctors. As a group they responded to our questions and demands with commendable promptness and thoroughness.

Special mention should be made of the help given us by Professor William G. Cochran of the Faculty of Arts and Sciences, Harvard College, and by Dr. Theodore Colton of the Department of Preventive Medicine of Harvard Medical School. Professor David D. Rutstein has given much advice and encouragement.

Miss Jean Haley and Miss Jan North, who have worked extensively on this manuscript, have greater reason than anyone else, perhaps, to take pleasure in seeing it completed. They have allowed us to revise it repeatedly with remarkably good humor.

During the period of planning, study execution, and first stages of analysis, Drs. Lyden and Geiger were members of the Department of Preventive Medicine, Harvard Medical School. Dr. Lyden was supported by a fellowship of the Health Information Foundation and Dr. Geiger was a Postdoctoral Research Fellow, Joint Program in Social Science in Medicine of the Department of Social Relations of Harvard University. Support for this study was provided by The Rockefeller Foundation.

# Contents

| | | |
|---|---|---|
| I | Why Study Doctors' Career Decisions? | 1 |
| II | Study Methods and Approach | 6 |
| III | Present Practice Circumstances | 19 |
| IV | Decisions about a Field of Practice | 48 |
| V | Hospital Training Decisions | 104 |
| VI | How the Graduates Viewed Their Medical Training | 186 |
| VII | Discussion and Conclusion | 212 |

References   241

Index   243

# Tables

1. Percentage distribution of doctors by present field of practice, 1961 — 20
2. Percentage distribution of doctors by amount of training they planned to obtain — 22
3. Percentage distribution of general practitioners by amount of training they planned to obtain — 24
4. Percentage distribution of doctors by age — 27
5. Percentage distribution by all doctors and doctors in certain fields of practice by age — 28
6. Percentage distribution of doctors by present type of practice relationship and type anticipated at peak of career — 30
7. Percentage distribution of general practitioners by present type of practice relationship and type anticipated at peak of career — 32
8. Percentage distribution of internists by present type of practice relationship and type anticipated at peak of career — 35
9. Percentage distribution of surgeons by present type of practice relationship and type anticipated at peak of career — 37
10. Percentage distribution of doctors by present location of practice — 38

TABLES

| | | |
|---|---|---|
| 11 | Percentage distribution of all groups by location of present practice | 40 |
| 12 | Percentage distribution of doctors by type of hospital appointment | 41 |
| 13 | Percentage distribution of doctors by 1961 taxable income | 43 |
| 14 | Percentage distribution of doctors reporting salary income as proportion of total medical income | 44 |
| 15 | Percentage distribution of doctors by value orientation and by field of practice | 47 |
| 16 | Percent of doctors strongly influenced in choice of a field of practice by factor and field of practice | 50 |
| 17 | Percentage distribution of doctors by father's education | 56 |
| 18 | Percentage distribution of employed persons by occpation and occupations of fathers of medical school graduates | 57 |
| 19 | Percentage distribution of doctors by place of birth | 62 |
| 20 | Percentage distribution of doctors by age at graduation | 65 |
| 21 | Percent of doctors reporting a major source of financial support for medical education by source | 67 |
| 22 | Percent of doctors reporting minor sources of financial support for medical education by source | 70 |
| 23 | Percentage distribution of doctors by yearly earnings while in medical school | 71 |

| | | |
|---|---|---|
| 24 | Percentage distribution of doctors by debt at graduation | 72 |
| 25 | Percent of doctors debt-free at conclusion of medical education | 74 |
| 26 | Percentage distribution of doctors by marital status | 78 |
| 27 | Percentage distribution of doctors by type of internship | 82 |
| 28 | Percentage distribution of doctors by field of practice and type of internship | 83 |
| 29 | Percentage distribution of doctors by hospital of internship | 85 |
| 30 | Percentage distribution of doctors by hospital of residency | 87 |
| 31 | Percent of doctors reporting 24 months or more residency training | 88 |
| 32 | Percent of doctors with residency and average duration of residency | 90 |
| 33 | Percent of doctors by field of practice and by composite MCAT score | 91 |
| 34 | Percentage distribution of doctors by field of practice and class rank | 93 |
| 35 | Percentage distribution of all doctors by time of final training decision and by field of practice | 97 |
| 36 | Percentage distribution of all doctors and general practitioners by amount of training decided upon | 98 |

| | | |
|---|---|---|
| 37 | Percent of doctors reporting encouragement in planning training by people influencing training beyond internship | 100 |
| 38 | Percent of doctors strongly influenced in choice of field of practice, by influential factor and type of internship | 106 |
| 39 | Percent of doctors strongly influenced in choice of field of practice by influential factor and by hospital of internship | 108 |
| 40 | Percent of doctors strongly influenced in choice of field of practice by influential factor and months of residency | 109 |
| 41 | Percent of doctors strongly influenced in choice of field of practice by influential factor and by class rank in thirds | 113 |
| 42 | Percentage distribution of doctors by hospital of internship and months of residency | 116 |
| 43 | Percent of doctors reporting residency by type of internship | 117 |
| 44 | Percentage distribution of 1954 graduates by MCAT scores | 119 |
| 45 | Percentage distribution of doctors by type of internship and by composite MCAT score | 119 |
| 46 | Percent of doctors by hospital of internship by composite MCAT score | 120 |

| | | |
|---|---|---|
| 47 | Percent of doctors with no residency by MCAT score | 121 |
| 48 | Percent of doctors by class rank with rotating or straight medical internship | 123 |
| 49 | Percent of doctors reporting major teaching hospital internship by class rank | 124 |
| 50 | Percent of doctors with residency training by class rank | 124 |
| 51 | Percentage distribution of doctors by father's education | 126 |
| 52 | Percentage distribution of doctors by father's education and hospital of internship | 127 |
| 53 | Percentage distribution of doctors by father's education and by hospital of residency | 129 |
| 54 | Percentage distribution of doctors of Eastern European and Eastern Mediterranean background by class rank | 130 |
| 55 | Percentage distribution of doctors by father's occupation and by hospital of internship, sons of craftsmen and all others | 133 |
| 56 | Percentage distribution of doctors by father's occupation and by hospital of residency, sons of craftsmen and all others | 135 |
| 57 | Percentage distribution of doctors by father's occupation, by months of residency | 136 |
| 58 | Percentage distribution of doctors born in large cities or in small towns by class rank | 137 |

| | TABLES | xiii |
|---|---|---|
| 59 | Percentage distribution of doctors reporting psychiatric residency and all others by place of birth | 139 |
| 60 | Percentage distribution of doctors by age at graduation and class rank | 140 |
| 61 | Percentage distribution of doctors by age at graduation and hospital of internship | 142 |
| 62 | Percentage distribution of doctors with residency and doctors with no residency by age at graduation | 144 |
| 63 | Percent of doctors by rotating or straight medical or surgical internships by major source of support | 147 |
| 64 | Percent of all doctors with major teaching hospital or other internships by major source of support | 149 |
| 65 | Percentage distribution of doctors reporting major support by parents and all others by months of residency | 150 |
| 66 | Percent of all doctors with major teaching and other hospital residency by major source of support | 151 |
| 67 | Percentage distribution of doctors by yearly earnings in medical school and by type of internship | 153 |
| 68 | Percentage distribution of doctors by yearly earnings in medical school by hospital of internship | 154 |
| 69 | Percentage distribution of doctors by yearly earnings while in medical school by hospital of residency | 156 |
| 70 | Percentage distribution of doctors by yearly earnings while in medical school by months of residency | 157 |

| | | |
|---|---|---|
| 71 | Percentage distribution of doctors with rotating and straight medical or surgical internships by amount of debt at graduation | 159 |
| 72 | Percentage distribution of doctors by debt at graduation and hospital of internship | 161 |
| 73 | Percentage distribution of doctors by residency or no residency and amount of debt at graduation | 162 |
| 74 | Percentage distribution of doctors by hospital of internship and marriage before entering medical school | 166 |
| 75 | Percentage distribution of doctors by marriage before medical school, by months of residency | 167 |
| 76 | Percentage distribution of doctors by MCAT score and class esteem ranking | 171 |
| 77 | Percentage distribution of doctors by class rank and class esteem ranking | 172 |
| 78 | Percentage distribution of class esteem leaders and other students by type of internship | 172 |
| 79 | Percent of doctors by class esteem ranking with major teaching hospital training | 173 |
| 80 | Percent of doctors by class esteem ranking with no residency | 173 |
| 81 | Percentage distribution of doctors by friendship group and by hospital of internship | 174 |
| 82 | Percent of doctors who were encouraged to obtain residency training by source of encouragement and by type of internship | 178 |

TABLES

| | | |
|---|---|---|
| 83 | Percent of doctors who were encouraged to obtain residency training by source of encouragement and by hospital of internship | 180 |
| 84 | Percent of doctors who were encouraged to obtain residency training by source of encouragement and hospital of residency | 182 |
| 85 | Percent of doctors who were encouraged to obtain residency by source of encouragement and by months of residency | 183 |
| 86 | Percent of doctors who were encouraged to obtain residency by source of encouragement and by class rank | 184 |
| 87 | Percent of doctors who were encouraged to obtain residency by source of encouragement and MCAT scores | 185 |
| 88 | Percentage distribution of doctors by dissatisfaction with medical education | 186 |
| 89 | Percentage distribution of doctors by dissatisfaction with medical education, general practitioners and all others | 188 |
| 90 | Percentage distribution of doctors by composite MCAT scores and dissatisfaction with medical education | 189 |
| 91 | Percentage distribution of doctors by hospital of internship and dissatisfaction with medical education | 190 |
| 92 | Percent of doctors with residency and no residency by dissatisfaction with medical education | 192 |

| | | |
|---|---|---|
| 93 | Percent of doctors dissatisfied with medical education, by months of residency | 193 |
| 94 | Percentage distribution of all doctors and general practitioners by major criticism of medical education | 194 |
| 95 | Percentage distribution of doctors stating criticism by composite MCAT scores and by major criticism | 196 |
| 96 | Percent of doctors dissatisfied with clinical training by academic rank | 197 |
| 97 | Percent of general practitioners and all other doctors dissatisfied with hospital training | 198 |
| 98 | Percentage distribution of doctors by opinion about hospital training by MCAT score | 199 |
| 99 | Percent of doctors with residency or no residency who were dissatisfied with hospital training | 199 |
| 100 | Percent of doctors dissatisfied with hospital training by months of residency | 200 |
| 101 | Percentage distribution of doctors reporting limitations of training by major responsible factor | 201 |
| 102 | Percentage distribution of general practitioners and all other doctors by frequency of curtailment of training, by responsible factor | 203 |
| 103 | Percentage distribution of doctors choosing the same or different training | 205 |
| 104 | Percent of doctors preferring the same internship as received by field of practice | 206 |

| | | |
|---|---|---|
| 105 | Percentage distribution of doctors by type of internship received and type preferred | 207 |
| 106 | Percentage distribution of doctors by preferred residency | 208 |
| 107 | Percentage distribution of doctors by preferred residency and by field of practice | 209 |
| 108 | Percentage distribution of doctors by preferred residency and by months of residency | 210 |

# I / Why Study Doctors' Career Decisions?

THE EVIDENCE indicates that most of the college students who intend to go to medical school ultimately obtain entry. These young people are from many diverse family, social, and educational backgrounds; when they enter medical school, they are forced into an educational program which, within each institution, is as uniform for all students as any program can be.

When these students leave medical school, they immediately pursue diverse programs of training. The internship and residency training programs they follow vary both in quality and length. Similarly, when they subsequently enter practice, they select many different and varied careers; these differences include place of practice, specialization or field, and the economic and professional organization of practice.

Unfortunately, there then appears still another kind of variation: in clinical skills, or—to characterize it more broadly—in the quality of practice. Numerous studies (and every physician's or medical educator's personal experience) demonstrate that doctors do vary in knowledge, skill, and the quality of their work. The several studies of general practitioners or other family doctors have all concluded that doctors' clinical skills are related to the amount of their clinical training, and suggest that, in general, longer hospital training is preferable to short training and that teaching-hospital experience is more effective preparation for practice than nonteaching-hospital experience. (6, 22, 23)

In short, then, a rather diverse group of students who undergo a very uniform medical school experience nevertheless maintain their diversity in their choice of further training and careers.

One reason for the importance of these choices is that they may have some influence on the quality of subsequent work. The present study is not concerned with whether or not doctors achieve clinical distinction. It is concerned with the differences between the doctors who prepare "well" for practice and those who do not. As part of this, it is concerned with the characteristics of the doctor which may influence him to obtain a "good" hospital training or that may influence him to enter practice with minimal preparation.

Clearly, the relationships between the length and quality of a doctor's training and his clinical skills are not simple. Medical students who rank high in their class obtain "better" internships and residencies than lower ranking students; yet there are also doctors of great skill whose training was short and in an undistinguished institution. There are also, undoubtedly, doctors who obtain excellent training but do not become clinically skilled. There is little doubt, however, that for the great majority of physicians, longer training is associated with greater clinical competence. Perhaps this greater competence reflects the training—or perhaps the doctors who select longer training are potentially more competent (or differ in some other significant way) to begin with.

For example, Peterson, Andrews, Spain, and Greenberg (23), as a sequel to the study of North Carolina general practitioners, studied another group of doctors with long clinical training. They found that as hospital training was prolonged, the doctors as a group became better and the variation among them became less. Perhaps the increased competence reflects the longer training; yet it is equally possible that the doctors who selected themselves for each additional year of training were more and more alike in certain respects, and potentially more skilled at the start.

Length of training is not the only significant variable; place of training may be important. Clute found, for example, that the clinical skills of general practitioners in practice were not related to the amount of nonteaching-hospital training they had received but that these skills were definitely related to length of training in teaching hospitals. Again, this may be a function of the training in the two kinds of hospitals, or of the men who select (or are selected for) this training, or both.

Thus, in studying the general question of the quality of physicians' performance, it becomes important to ask: Who chooses longer training and who chooses less? Why? Who chooses teaching-hospital training and who does not? Why? What are the roles of personal variables—intellectual, financial, family background, and the like—in these choices? What other factors influence them?

Until recently, relatively little attention has been given these questions. In contrast, much attention and study have been given to the selection of medical students, a question of importance, of course, but one which should not be allowed to obscure the basic concern of medical education: the competence of the graduate physician. A few studies have been concerned with what happens to the students after they leave medical school, as exemplified by studies in which students were asked what type of practice they expected to enter. The many specialty boards, with their important power of certification, are further evidence of the importance attached to residency training. Nevertheless, the great variability in the available hospital training programs and the freedom with which the medical school graduate can select among them—freedom which is not to be criticized as such—results in the unfortunate situation that many doctors obtain poor hospital training that gives them little help in becoming skilled doctors.

It is, therefore, important that the choices that the doctor makes about his training and about his practice be examined. Such an examination must be made with full realization that a student's choices will be modified by his material and intellectual resources, as well as those of his family; furthermore, the complexity of the factors which influence these choices should not be neglected. The medical students may attend a public or a private medical school; one that is large or small; a school with a long tradition and a wealth of faculty or another that has recently been formed. Attendance at one type of medical school may lead easily into a hospital training program that is seldom open to the students of other schools.

In this study the medical student, the school, and the hospital have been examined to see how each is associated with the doctors' preparation for practice and selection of a field of practice. Naturally, there was interest in finding any facts that might be of predictive value. Is there, for example, any type of medical school student who is more likely than any other to prepare himself well for practice? Such student characteristics were not the only subject of interest. It was hoped that it would be possible to determine whether the circumstances which limit the preparation of some doctors are remediable.

Good clinical training is not the only determinant of good medical care. Medical care insurance, hospitals, and other facilities are also necessary. However, competent doctors are the most essential single element. Since the measurement of a doctor's competence requires difficult and exhaustive direct studies of practice and is therefore not practical on a large scale, this study has concerned itself with the doctor's hospital training. Although training is not as good a measure of the outcome of the medical education process as is competence, the evidence from direct studies that training and competence are strongly related justifies our use of training as the critical characteristic under investigation.

# II / Study Methods and Approach

THE PURPOSE of this study is to determine the factors which influence some doctors to obtain longer and better training and others to obtain shorter and poorer preparation for practice. Since certain types of practice, such as neurosurgery, are almost invariably associated with long periods of training in teaching hospitals, whereas other fields are associated with extremely variable periods and types of hospital training, the question "training for what?" is implicitly part of the study purpose.

The approach we have taken is to consider first the present professional and family circumstances of the doctors included in the study. Next we examine the respondents' social and economic backgrounds, and relate these to the choice of a field of specialty practice. The respondents' academic performance in medical school and their subsequent hospital training are then related to their social and economic backgrounds and circumstances in medical school. Finally, we consider how the respondents evaluate the medical education and hospital training they received. This evaluation includes: whether they received as much training or the type of training they now believe they needed, and if not, why not; what shortcomings they now perceive in the educational process they experienced, and what they feel should be done about these deficiencies; and in retrospect, how they would restructure their training experience if they had a chance to do it over.

*Selection of Population Sample*

Most empirical studies of the training and career decisions of doctors have been based on samples of medical students. The

## STUDY METHODS AND APPROACH

student has been asked to indicate what additional training he expects to receive and what practice relationships he expects to enter into after graduation.(2, 13, 19) The difficulty with this approach is that many medical students may not yet have made decisions about these questions, and even those who have may well change their minds as the result of circumstances they encounter during their hospital training. For this reason, we decided that it would be more useful to approach doctors who had already completed their hospital training and had made at least tentative decisions about their specialty and practice relationships.

The decision to study recent medical school graduates was made for several reasons. The doctors who attended medical school during World War II did so under very unusual circumstances that have little relevance to what might be regarded as normal. On the other hand, the postwar period saw a vast expansion in the available internship and residency programs and a marked increase in inclination among doctors to pursue extensive training before going into practice. The experiences of the doctors who finished medical school before the United States entered World War II are, therefore, not relevant to the problems of today. In questioning doctors about events that occurred during their internship and residency, it is clearly desirable to tax memory as little as possible; this provided another justification for the limitation of the study to men who had graduated recently. Since planning for the study began in 1960, we decided to include 1954 graduates, assuming that almost all of these men would be in practice seven years after the event. It was expected that men graduating in this year would be more representative of normal medical school output than in the earlier postwar period when a large proportion of medical students were veterans and, therefore, both older and recipients of support under the G.I. Bill. The 1950 classes were selected as the second group of study for several reasons. Since they were removed by four years in time from the 1954 class, they might be sufficiently remote and sufficiently different to show any trends that were developing with respect to hospital training and distribution between different fields of practice. Examination of this group was expected to yield information on the extent to which financial aid to veterans affected either the length or the type of hospital training pursued.

All the graduates of the classes of 1950 and 1954 in a limited number of medical schools were studied instead of nationwide random sampling for several reasons. The group of students who go through a given medical school together have a common experience. Because of this uniformity of educational experience individual student or family characteristics should have greater meaning. Furthermore, any possible influence of students upon one another can be measured best under circumstances where information on entire classes is available. Finally, this method permits examination of the school itself (or type of school) as a variable with possible influence on students' choices.

*Selection of Schools*

The medical schools studied were selected on the basis of characteristics important to the goals of this investigation; varied data contributed to this decision. There is ample evidence from studies of Dickenson and others (10, 29) that the graduates of publicly supported and privately supported medical schools differ in their tendency to enter general or specialty practice or teaching and research. Public and private schools also have different problems in selecting medical students. Moreover, within the publicly supported and privately supported groups certain

# STUDY METHODS AND APPROACH

schools have, for years, tended to produce more teachers and research workers, others have tended to produce specialists, and still others to produce chiefly general practitioners. Schools of all three types were included in the sample. Thirdly, it was felt that the size of the medical school might have an influence upon students and hence upon their subsequent training. Lastly, it was reasoned that geographic location of medical schools could not be ignored even though there is no evidence that location, per se, has an effect upon a medical school's output.

Church related and predominantly Negro medical schools were excluded because they would have expanded the study beyond a size judged to be feasible. Although both of these groups are small, giving them adequate representation would have necessitated unduly heavy sampling within each category.

Another consideration in selecting the schools was the possibility of comparisons with the longitudinal studies being conducted by the Association of American Medical Colleges (AAMC), which has been following the careers of graduates from twenty-eight medical schools since 1956. The institutions which are the subject of this report are mostly included in the AAMC study; a few are not.

Twelve schools were selected to provide a balance of the characteristics enumerated above. The number of schools by categories for each of the four characteristics are as follows.

| Ownership | Number of schools | Size | Number of schools |
|---|---|---|---|
| Public | 6 | Large | 5 |
| Private | 6 | Small | 7 |
| *Traditional output* | | *Location* | |
| General practitioner | 5 | East | 4 |
| Specialty | 4 | Midwest | 3 |
| Teaching | | South | 3 |
| and research | 3 | West | 2 |

A total interview sample of about 2000 doctors was estimated as necessary to permit breakdowns by various types of practice, school, and other characteristics. A study of this size was also deemed to be feasible. The 1950 and 1954 graduates of the twelve selected medical schools totaled 1887, a reasonably close approximation of the sample size desired.

*Questionnaire Design and Administration*

To make feasible a study involving doctors from twelve medical schools from all parts of the United States, a mailed questionnaire was employed. Since doctors are characteristically very busy people and a considerable amount of information was necessary from each respondent, a questionnaire was developed that was thorough but still could be completed in a reasonable length of time. Where possible, questions were phrased so that they could be answered by a check mark; other questions were phrased in such a way that the doctor could answer with one or two words. The questionnaires were pretested on a number of practitioners to eliminate, so far as possible, ambiguity or bias in wording.*

To insure a high response rate, each of the twelve schools selected for inclusion in the study was visited by a member of the study staff. The purpose and nature of the study was explained and each school's cooperation and support was elicited. The dean of each school agreed to send a letter to all of his 1950 and 1954 graduates urging them to cooperate in responding to the questionnaire.

Assiduous follow-up of nonrespondents resulted in the ultimate return of questionnaires by 1771 doctors—an overall 94

* A copy of the questionnaire may be obtained from the authors.

## STUDY METHODS AND APPROACH 11

percent response rate. Considerable data was available on the nonresponders and is included in many of the tables of this report. For example, all of the nonresponders could be categorized by class rank, and the composite Medical College Admission Test (MCAT) scores were known for most of the 1954 graduates in the nonresponder group. Further, the place and type of practice could be determined for some. The small size of the nonresponder group precludes any substantial bias, due to lack of response, in the general findings of the study.

Most of the nonresponders simply chose not to fill in the questionnaire. A few did not receive the questionnaire because they could not be reached despite an extended search for their current address and location. The available information does not indicate any systematic selection of nonresponders.

The percentage of graduates from each school who returned the questionnaires are as follows.

| *Public Schools* | 1950 | 1954 | Combined |
|---|---|---|---|
| A | 86 | 95 | |
| B | 98 | 94 | |
| C | 84 | 94 | |
| D | 86 | 98 | |
| E | 93 | 93 | |
| F | 88 | 98 | |
| All Public Schools | 89 | 95 | 93 |
| *Private Schools* | | | |
| A' | 95 | 92 | |
| B' | 86 | 98 | |
| C' | 91 | 100 | |
| D' | 93 | 99 | |
| E' | 91 | 95 | |
| F' | 98 | 96 | |
| All Private Schools | 93 | 97 | 95 |
| All Schools | 91 | 96 | 94 |

The numbers of respondents in the four groups were as follows.

|  | 1950 | 1954 | Total |
|---|---|---|---|
| Six Public Schools | 334 | 498 | 832 |
| Six Private Schools | 430 | 509 | 939 |
| Total |  |  | 1,771 |

The returned questionnaires constituted 15 and 14 percent of all graduates of United States medical schools in 1950 and 1954 respectively.

A study of the returned questionnaires showed that they were completed with commendable care. The frequent addition of explanatory notes and very occasional criticisms of the questionnaire technique itself were taken as further evidence of the conscientiousness of the doctors in providing information.

*Data Analysis*

Coded responses to all questions in the questionnaire were transferred to punched cards and answers were tabulated by private or public schools and by year of graduation. Tables were prepared to show how the responses on each training and career decision variable were related to the responses given to every other pertinent question in the questionnaire. Most data reported in this volume will be presented in terms of such contingency tables. This was done so that any characteristic that proved to differentiate the schools in terms of their graduates' decisions about training or careers could be held constant for purpose of analysis.

Two questions attempted to elicit the "value orientation" of each respondent, that is, the criteria he felt to be most important in identifying a good doctor or a good medical student. The scale originated by James Coleman, Elihu Katz, and Herbert

STUDY METHODS AND APPROACH 13

Menzel(8) was utilized, adjusting the wording to fit the context of this study.

Analysis of variance was conducted to relate various school characteristics (for example, public or private, size) to (1) traditional output (graduates' distribution by fields of practice—the percentage distribution of general practitioners, specialists, and teachers and research workers); and (2) the various characteristics of the training obtained by graduates—length of residency, type of residency hospital, and so forth. The size and location of the medical school was found to have no measurable effect upon its graduates' hospital training or selection of a field of practice. Greater variance was found between the public and private medical school graduates in both 1950 and 1954 than was found within either the public or private groups. As the accompanying tabulations show, the difference between the public and private school graduates was marked and consistent when examined by proportion of graduates in general practice and length of residency. (P usually = <.001.) When schools were classified by their traditional output, the differences were not as great or consistent.

VARIANCE ANALYSIS BY FIELD OF PRACTICE

Public-Private, 1950

| Source | Sums of squares | Degree of freedom | Mean of square |
|---|---|---|---|
| Between | 1026.75 | 1 | 1026.75 |
| Within | 389.46 | 10 | 38.95 |
| Total | 1416.21 | 11 | |

Traditional Output, 1950

| Source | Sums of squares | Degree of freedom | Mean of square |
|---|---|---|---|
| Between | 0.2183 | 2 | 0.1093 |
| Within | 0.0890 | 9 | 0.0099 |
| Total | 0.3073 | 11 | |

Public-Private, 1954

| Source | Sums of squares | Degree of freedom | Mean of square |
|---|---|---|---|
| Between | 1587.00 | 1 | 1587.00 |
| Within | 648.52 | 10 | 64.86 |
| Total | 2235.52 | 11 | |

Traditional Output, 1954

| Source | Sums of squares | Degree of freedom | Mean of square |
|---|---|---|---|
| Between | 0.3148 | 2 | 0.1574 |
| Within | 0.1111 | 9 | 0.0123 |
| Total | 0.4259 | 11 | |

## VARIANCE ANALYSIS BY LENGTH OF RESIDENCY TRAINING

Public-Private, 1950

| Source | Sums of squares | Degree of freedom | Mean of square |
|---|---|---|---|
| Between | 7.5209 | 1 | 7.5209 |
| Within | 3.3733 | 10 | 0.3373 |
| Total | 10.8942 | 11 | |

Traditional Output, 1950

| Source | Sums of squares | Degree of freedom | Mean of square |
|---|---|---|---|
| Between | 5.4756 | 2 | 2.7378 |
| Within | 5.4186 | 9 | 0.6021 |
| Total | 10.8942 | 11 | |

Public-Private, 1954

| Source | Sums of squares | Degree of freedom | Mean of square |
|---|---|---|---|
| Between | 9.8827 | 1 | 9.8827 |
| Within | 5.0280 | 10 | 0.5028 |
| Total | 14.9107 | 11 | |

Traditional Output, 1954

| Source | Sums of squares | Degree of freedom | Mean of square |
|---|---|---|---|
| Between | 6.7901 | 2 | 3.3950 |
| Within | 8.1206 | 9 | 0.9023 |
| Total | 14.9107 | 11 | |

On the basis of these results, it was obvious that the most important *school* characteristic to hold constant in analyzing the data was the public versus private character of the institution. Therefore, all data reported in this study are presented in terms of public and private school respondents.

Although our tables list "teaching and research" as a distinct group, doctors who are reported as engaged in teaching or research may also be trained as internists, surgeons, psychiatrists, or other specialists. Virtually all of the pertinent tables were re-examined after redistribution of the clinically trained numbers of the teaching-research group among the appropriate specialties; since the effect of this redistribution was negligible, the teaching-research group has been maintained throughout the volume.

### *Tests of Significance and Interpretation of Results*

Statistical tests of significance have been employed in this book as a guide to the reader in interpreting results relative to the magnitude of school-to-school variation. Since the selection

## STUDY METHODS AND APPROACH

of schools for this study was purposive and not at random, in the strictest sense the usual interpretation of statistical tests of significance is not appropriate.

However, the twelve schools selected accounted for 15 percent of all medical school graduates for 1950 and 1954, which is an appreciable proportion. Furthermore, as we have indicated, the sample cuts across the important variables of geographic location; public-private status; traditional output of general practitioners, specialists, or teacher-researchers; and size. Although there may be several respects in which the schools selected might be somewhat atypical or unrepresentative of all medical schools, for the most part we have obtained a wide spectrum of characteristics, insuring against an extreme form of selection for our sample.

For this reason we have calculated standard errors and applied tests of significance as if our sample were one selected at random. We have been extremely cautious in the interpretation of statistically significant differences. Hence, it is extremely unlikely that results labeled "statistically significant" can be attributed to the purposive sample selection.

The tests of significance employed involved comparisons of proportions. Where tests were used, the variances of the proportions involved were calculated by treating schools as "clusters" with 100 percent enumeration within the cluster. These variances were determined following a procedure outlined by Cochran.(7)

To compare two proportions, $p_1$ and $p_2$, the critical ratio (CR) consisting of

$$CR = \frac{p_1 - p_2}{\sqrt{(\text{Variance of } p_1) + (\text{Variance of } p_2)}}$$

was calculated.

To examine a trend in proportions—for example, to test for a trend by class rank—a weighted regression coefficient was obtained, the weights being the inverses of the variances. The notation is as follows.

| Third of class | Lower | Middle | Upper |
|---|---|---|---|
| $x_i$ | 0 | 1 | 2 |
| Proportion with ($P_i$) desired characteristic | $P_0$ | $P_1$ | $P_2$ |
| Variance of $P_i$ | $\sigma_0^2$ | $\sigma_1^2$ | $\sigma_2^2$ |
| Weight ($w_i$) | $w_0 = 1/\sigma_0^2$ | $w_1 = 1/\sigma_1^2$ | $w_2 = 1/\sigma_2^2$ |

The regression coefficient, then, is

$$b = \frac{\Sigma w_i x_i p_i - (\Sigma w_i x_i)(\Sigma w_i p_i)/(\Sigma w_i)}{\Sigma w_i x_i - (\Sigma w_i x_i)^2/(\Sigma w_i)}.$$

The standard error of the regression coefficient is

$$SE(b) = 1/\sqrt{\Sigma w_i t_i^2 - (\Sigma w_i t_i)^2/(\Sigma w_i)},$$

and a critical ratio of

$$CR = b/SE(b)$$

was determined.

Critical ratios exceeding 2 were labeled significant and correspond roughly to the 5 percent level. Critical ratios exceeding 3 were labeled highly significant and correspond roughly to the 0.1 percent level.

## Definition of Terms

In the presentation of data derived from the questionnaires, a number of terms acquire specific meanings. Since almost all of the data will be broken down by year of graduation and by the character of the medical school attended, whether public or private, "groups" will be used quite commonly to designate the four major divisions: the 1950 private school graduates, the 1954 private school graduates, the 1950 public school graduates, and the 1954 public school graduates.

"Percentage distribution," as used in most of the table headings, indicates that all of the doctors studied are included in the denominator. In these tables the various percentages will normally total 100. "Percent" in table headings is used where multiple answers to a single question were possible or where only part of the total group of doctors found the question applicable. In both of these instances the total percent is usually more or less than 100.

"No response" is used in tables to show the proportion of physicians who did not answer a specific question; it does not include those who failed to return the questionnaire. Since this category was very small it has been omitted from some tables, especially those in which two types of nonresponse complicated the presentation without adding essential information.

In all tables the number of doctors used as the base for calculation is the number in parenthesis. Its location indicates the column or line to which it is applicable. In some instances the base for calculation will vary slightly from table to table due to inclusion or omission of the nonresponders. Since each question may lack responses the different tables dealing with a particular variable may show slightly different numbers used as a base.

"Type of internship" is used throughout the text and in tables to indicate whether an internship program was rotating, straight service, or mixed. Straight medical or surgical internships are normally listed solely as "surgical" or "medical."

"Hospital of internship" refers to the teaching characteristics of the institution. In most tables the hospitals are broken down into "major teaching" and "other." In a few tables in which the minor teaching hospitals are included as a separate group, it will be seen that they are not characteristically different from the nonteaching hospitals with accredited internships or residencies. It is for this reason that these two groups have been lumped throughout the text as "other."

# III / Present Practice Circumstances

THE RESPONSES to our questionnaire will enable us to examine the doctor's decisions about his career—field of practice, type of practice, type and amount of professional training, and the like—in relation to many of the variables which may have influenced these decisions. First, our task is to examine in broad terms the characteristics and demography of this sample of physicians. In 1961, at the time they responded to our questionnaire, what was their distribution with regard to field of practice: general practitioner, internist, surgeon, pediatrician, or other fields? Were they board-certified or not? What was their age distribution? Were they in solo practice, group practice, partnership, or hospital practice, and did they anticipate any change? Where were their offices located? Did they have a hospital appointment? What was their distribution with regard to income? What were their family and marital circumstances?

*Field of Practice*

Table 1 displays the percentage distribution of 1950 and 1954 public and private school graduates by field of practice. A striking feature in both years is the much greater proportion of public than private school graduates in general practice: 35 percent versus 14 percent in 1950 (CR 4.4), and 33 percent versus only 8 percent in 1954 (CR 5.4). Conversely, the proportion of specialists in private schools was significantly higher than that in public schools in both 1950 and 1954. The critical ratio of the public-

TABLE 1. Percentage distribution of doctors by present field of practice, type of school, and year of graduation, 1961

| | Public | | Private | |
| Field of practice | 1950 | 1954 | 1950 | 1954 |
|---|---|---|---|---|
| General practice | 35 | 33 | 14 | 8 |
| Medicine* | 16 | 15 | 17 | 21 |
| Surgery | 15 | 13 | 22 | 24 |
| Pediatrics | 4 | 5 | 8 | 8 |
| Obstetrics-gynecology | 4 | 6 | 6 | 5 |
| Psychiatry | 7 | 7 | 8 | 7 |
| Teaching-research | 6 | 8 | 14 | 17 |
| Other | 13 | 13 | 9 | 10 |
| Not in practice | 1 | 1 | 2 | 1 |
| | (334) | (498) | (430) | (509) |

*Medicine=internal medicine

private school difference in the proportion of specialists was 4.7 for 1950 and 3.2 for 1954.*

* See above, pages 16–18 for a definition of terms used in the tables. For a full explanation of the critical ratio (CR) and its use in these data, see pages 14–16. A CR exceeding 2.0 corresponds roughly to the 5 percent level (0.05); a CR exceeding 3.0 corresponds roughly to the 0.1 percent level (0.001). Thus, a CR of 4.4 is significant at a level well beyond one in a thousand. The reader may note that the differences between doctor classes are from time to time described as not significant despite percentage differences that appear to be substantial. Reference to the formulas and explanation of the critical ratio calculations will make it clear that variance within a category (for example, school-by-school variance among private school internists expressing strong patient orientation) is also an important factor, and that high variance will lower the critical ratio.

Although the overall proportion of general practitioners decreased from 1950 to 1954, the absolute number increased by 15 percent, from 177 in 1950 to 204 in 1954. This increase in absolute number was produced entirely by the public schools however, for they graduated 116 general practitioners in 1950 and 164 in 1954, while the corresponding private school output actually fell from 61 to 40.

The output of internists, in contrast, was relatively stable, except for a slight increase from 1950 to 1954 in the proportion of internists who graduated from private schools. There is no substantial public-private school difference in the proportion of graduates who chose internal medicine as their field of practice.

If general practitioners and physicians practicing internal medicine are grouped together as real or potential "family doctors," the public schools again produce the higher proportions: 51 percent of all public school graduates in 1950 are accounted for by these two rubrics, as opposed to 31 percent of private school graduates, and 48 percent as opposed to 29 percent for 1954. The combined output of possible family doctors in 1950 was 41 percent of the total; since this figure includes doctors whose practices are described as cardiology, gastroenterology, and many other limited subspecialties, these figures overstate the proportions of actual family doctors.

The proportion of graduates becoming surgeons is relatively stable from 1950 to 1954. In both years the private schools produced a higher proportion of surgeons. A striking difference appears between public and private schools in the output of graduates entering teaching and research in both 1950 and 1954, with private schools producing significantly more teachers and researchers. Although the differences in percentage displayed in Table 1 do not, at first inspection, seem extreme, the critical ratios were 2.0 for 1950 and 2.2 for 1954.

In summary, Table 1 suggests great stability, from 1950 to 1954, in the field of practice choices of public school graduates, with one in every three entering general practice. In 1950 only one in seven private school graduates entered general practice, and by 1954 this had declined to less than one in twelve, with a corresponding increase in those selecting internal medicine, surgery, and academic medicine. Overall, the proportion of general practitioners and of potential family doctors declined slightly.

*Training and Certification*

All respondents, in outlining their medical education, were asked, "How much training did you finally decide to obtain?" Their answers, grouped by year and type of school, are presented in Table 2. Again, there is a striking public-private school dif-

TABLE 2. Percentage distribution of doctors by amount of training they planned to obtain, by type of school and year of graduation

| Amount of training planned | Public | | Private | |
|---|---|---|---|---|
| | 1950 | 1954 | 1950 | 1954 |
| Internship only | 29 | 23 | 7 | 4 |
| Partial residency | 11 | 11 | 12 | 8 |
| Certification | 60 | 65 | 80 | 88 |
| No response | 1 | 0 | 0 | 1 |
| | (334) | (498) | (430) | (509) |

ference. From four to nearly six times as many public school graduates in 1950 (CR 9.0) and 1954 (CR 5.1) planned to obtain internship only. There is a corresponding and significant excess in the proportion of private school graduates planning to obtain complete residency training and specialty certification in 1950 (CR 4.1) and 1954 (CR 4.6). The proportion of those planning partial residency training was similar in public and private schools and did not change substantially from 1950 to 1954. A time trend is evident: in both public and private schools the proportion planning internship only declined slightly from 1950 to 1954, and the proportion planning certification increased correspondingly.

It should be emphasized that many of the respondents—especially those from the 1954 classes—were describing their plans or intentions in answering this question.

A few physicians among all the doctors who had intended to obtain residency training did not. Thirty and twenty-five percent of the 1950 and 1954 public school graduates actually terminated their hospital training with an internship. The corresponding figures for the private school graduates were 9 and 4 percent. The intent to obtain certification and its actual achievement showed a greater disparity. By 1962, 35 percent of the public and 54 percent of the private school graduates of 1950 were certified. The distribution of this cohort by year of certification showed that very few were still being certified in the years immediately preceding 1962; it is therefore apparent that little change is to be anticipated in these percentages. Twenty-four and thirty-six percent of the public and private graduates of 1954 were certified by 1962 in contrast with 65 and 88 percent, respectively, who stated this intention. In this cohort, certification was still being obtained, so the figures are not complete.

If we examine the training plans of general practitioners only (Table 3), major differences between public and private school graduates are once again evident. In both 1950 and 1954 from two thirds to three fourths of the general practitioners graduating from public schools planned to obtain only an internship. Though the proportion planning a partial residence increased from 22 to 32 percent, only a very few planned sufficient further training for certification. In contrast, only about one third of the future general practitioners graduating from private schools planned to limit themselves to internship training; the majority in both 1950 and 1954 planned a partial residency, though the proportion planning to obtain certification decreased from 15 to 10 percent.

The public and private school general practitioner graduates were significantly different with respect to their training decisions. For example, the difference in proportions of respondents planning only an internship were highly significant in both 1950 (CR 9.8) and in 1954 (3.2). Similarly, the different proportions of public and private school graduates planning partial or full

TABLE 3. Percentage distribution of general practitioners by amount of training they planned to obtain, by type of school and year of graduation

| Amount of training planned | Public | | Private | |
| --- | --- | --- | --- | --- |
| | 1950 | 1954 | 1950 | 1954 |
| Internship | 76 | 64 | 28 | 33 |
| Partial residency | 22 | 32 | 57 | 58 |
| Certification in a specialty | 2 | 4 | 15 | 10 |
| | (116) | (164) | (61) | (40) |

residency (sufficient for certification) were all significant (CR range from 2.3 to 5.4) except for 1954 graduates planning certification. The numbers in this last strata were very small. The private school graduates who entered general practice had definitely more ambitious plans for training than those who graduated from public medical schools.

When general practitioners are compared with all other physicians with regard to planned amount of training, huge differences appear. For example, among 1950 public school graduates the difference between general practitioners and others planning to obtain internship only was overwhelming (CR 23.7); the same is true among 1954 public school graduates (CR 20.7). Among private school graduates the differences between general practitioners and other doctors planning to obtain internship only were also significant, but not at such extremely high levels (CR 5.7 in 1950, 3.3 in 1954).

Conversely, very large and significant differences occur between the percentages of general practitioners and of all other doctors planning complete residency training and specialty certification. Among public school graduates the CR of this difference was more than 45 in 1950 and 27.0 in 1954, while for private school graduates the percentage of general practitioners who planned certification was also significantly lower than that of all other doctors in both years (CR 13.8 in 1950 and 14.6 in 1954).

The same is true of general practioners versus all other doctors planning partial residency training, with significantly fewer general practioners planning to obtain such training among public school graduates (CR 4.8 and 10.0) and private school graduates (CR 9.2 and 6.1) in the two years.

The public and private school graduates who were not general practitioners did not differ significantly insofar as their decisions about training were concerned. The differences between public and private schools illustrated in Table 2 were thus due almost entirely to the differences in proportions of graduates entering general practice and to differences between the general practitioners graduating from the two types of schools.

### Age

The age of the respondents may be described in several ways: as age at entering medical school, age at graduation, or age at the time of the study (1961). The nature of the sample affects each measure: the fact that the class of 1950 included many World War II veterans whose education had been delayed by military service, and thus were older, adds to the anticipated differential between the classes of 1950 and 1954.

The age in 1961 of respondents is shown in Table 4; again a difference between public and private schools is evident. Forty-seven percent of the 1950 public school graduates were twenty-nine years or older at the time of graduation (that is, forty years or older in 1961), compared to 36 percent of the private school graduates. This difference is not significant. In the 1954 classes, however, 22 percent of the public school graduates, compared with 10 percent of the private school graduates, were twenty-nine years or older at the time of graduation (that is, 36 years or older in 1961). This is a significant difference (CR 2.9).

In both the public and private schools the proportion of older graduates in the 1950 classes was far higher than in the 1954 classes. These differences, which are significant (CR 5.4 for 1950–1954 public school difference, and CR 6.2 for 1950–1954 private school difference), are undoubtedly due to the large number of veterans in the class of 1950.

TABLE 4. Percentage distribution of doctors by age (1961) by year of graduation and type of school

| 1950 | | | 1954 | | |
| Age | Public | Private | Age | Public | Private |
| --- | --- | --- | --- | --- | --- |
| 42- | 29 | 16 | 38- | 10 | 3 |
| 40-41 | 18 | 20 | 36-37 | 12 | 7 |
| 38-39 | 19 | 19 | 34-35 | 28 | 26 |
| 36-37 | 17 | 22 | 32-33 | 42 | 50 |
| 34-35 | 15 | 18 | 31- | 7 | 12 |
| 32-33 | 2 | 1 | | | |
| No response | 1 | 3 | No response | 1 | 2 |
| | (334) | (430) | | (498) | (509) |

These relationships are also evident in Table 5, in which the age in 1961 was used to divide the classes of 1950 and 1954. When field of practice is considered, it is immediately evident that, in both time periods and in both groups of schools, general practitioners are substantially older than their classmates. Thus, of the 1950 graduating classes 47 and 38 were forty and older in 1961—but 58 and 57 percent of the 1950 public and private graduates who became general practitioners were in this age group. Graduates who became internists did not vary in any consistent manner from all doctors, but surgeons and those in teaching and research had higher percentages in the "under forty" category. The increased age of general practitioners is even more striking in the 1954 class. While only 50 and 37 percent of all the public and private 1954 graduates were thirty-four and

TABLE 5. Percentage distribution of all doctors and doctors in certain fields of practice by age in 1961

| Age | Public | | | | Private | | | |
|---|---|---|---|---|---|---|---|---|
| | All doctors | General practice | Surgery | Teaching and research | All doctors | General practice | Surgery | Teaching and research |
| | | | | 1950 | | | | |
| 40- | 47 | 58 | 32 | 42 | 38 | 57 | 35 | 22 |
| -39 | 53 | 42 | 68 | 58 | 62 | 43 | 65 | 78 |
| | (332) | (116) | (50) | (19) | (415) | (58) | (91) | (58) |
| | | | | 1954 | | | | |
| 34- | 50 | 67 | 38 | 38 | 37 | 61 | 30 | 27 |
| -33 | 50 | 33 | 62 | 62 | 63 | 39 | 70 | 73 |
| | (491) | (163) | (63) | (37) | (499) | (38) | (121) | (84) |

over in 1961, 67 and 61 percent of the public and private school graduates who became general practitioners were in this age category. Those in surgery and teaching and research were represented most heavily in the "thirty-three or younger" group, while those in other specialties followed the total distribution. Apparently, the tendency for older students to enter general practice was not a postwar phenomenon; if anything, this tendency was diluted by the presence of many older students in the 1950 class and appeared somewhat more strikingly in 1954. The differences between the general practitioners and other physicians were all significant (general practitioners versus others: public, 1950, CR = 2.0, and 1954, CR = 4.0; private, 1950, CR = 3.3 and 1954, CR = 2.0). The differences between the smaller groups of surgeons and teachers and researchers and the corresponding "other" groups—"other, not surgeon" and "other, not teacher-researcher"—reached significant levels only occasionally. Between 1950 and 1954 the age distribution of those entering medical practice shifted toward the younger side; it is for this reason that different scales are used in the tables for 1950 and 1954.

## Type of Practice

Respondents were asked to describe their current type of practice—solo, group, partnership, hospital, or other—and, in addition, were asked to state the type of practice they anticipated at the peaks of their careers. Table 6 presents the responses for graduates of public schools and private schools in 1950 and 1954.

Perhaps the most striking feature is the anticipated decline of solo practice. While solo practice accounts for almost half of both public and private school graduates of 1950, only about

TABLE 6. Percentage distribution of doctors by present type of practice relationship, 1961, and type anticipated at peak of career, by type of school and year of graduation

| Practice relationship | 1950 | | | | 1954 | | | |
|---|---|---|---|---|---|---|---|---|
| | Public | | Private | | Public | | Private | |
| | Now | Anticipated | Now | Anticipated | Now | Anticipated | Now | Anticipated |
| Solo | 48 | 34 | 48 | 34 | 36 | 25 | 30 | 25 |
| Group | 15 | 19 | 10 | 12 | 16 | 23 | 11 | 18 |
| Hospital | 12 | 7 | 14 | 12 | 21 | 9 | 32 | 17 |
| Partnership | 18 | 26 | 14 | 22 | 18 | 31 | 12 | 21 |
| Other | 6 | 6 | 11 | 10 | 7 | 6 | 13 | 11 |
| No response | 1 | 8 | 3 | 9 | 1 | 5 | 2 | 8 |
| | (334) | | (430) | | (498) | | (509) | |

one third of the classes of 1954 currently practice alone. Furthermore, nearly one third of all current solo practitioners plan to change to another type of practice at the peaks of their careers, so that ultimately solo practice will account for only about 35 percent of the class of 1950 and about 25 percent of the 1954 graduates. There is no difference between public and private schools with regard to solo practice (current or anticipated) in the 1950 cohort, and only a slight difference in 1954.

There is no major public-private difference in the frequency of partnership practice—current or anticipated in 1950—and the upward trend from "current" to "anticipated" status in this category is similar in the two groups. In 1954, however, partnership is more common among public than private school graduates with respect to both current and anticipated status. This may be due at least in part to the fact that hospital practice (including many individuals still in training) is a much more common current status in 1954 than in 1950. In 1954 the private school graduates' current practice and anticipated practice involves the hospital more frequently than is the case with public school graduates (CR 2.3).

Group practice shows relative stability. It is somewhat more favored by public than by private school graduates, both currently and in terms of future planning, and it shows some increase from 1950 to 1954.

When we examine these current and anticipated choices by field of practice, it becomes clear that general practitioners constitute the great stronghold of solo practice, both now and in the future, though even in this group there is a decline in solo practice from 1950 to 1954 and from current to anticipated choices. As Table 7 shows, an absolute majority of general practitioners in 1950, and a bare majority in the 1954 class are currently

TABLE 7. Percentage distribution of general practitioners by present type of practice relationship, 1961, and type anticipated at peak of career, by type of school and year of graduation

| Practice relationship | 1950 | | | | 1954 | | | |
|---|---|---|---|---|---|---|---|---|
| | Public | | Private | | Public | | Private | |
| | Now | Anticipated | Now | Anticipated | Now | Anticipated | Now | Anticipated |
| Solo | 60 | 47 | 66 | 54 | 46 | 30 | 55 | 38 |
| Group | 10 | 16 | 8 | 11 | 18 | 25 | 13 | 23 |
| Hospital | 1 | 0 | 0 | 0 | 4 | 4 | 3 | 0 |
| Partnership | 26 | 27 | 25 | 28 | 28 | 30 | 20 | 20 |
| Other | 2 | 3 | 2 | 3 | 3 | 2 | 8 | 10 |
| No response | 1 | 8 | 0 | 3 | 1 | 9 | 3 | 10 |
| | (116) | | (61) | | (164) | | (40) | |

(1961) in solo practice. About half of the 1950 graduate general practitioners and about one third of the 1954 graduates plan to be in solo practice at the peaks of their careers. Solo practice, both present and anticipated, is somewhat more favored by private school than by public school graduates in both years, but the difference is not significant. Among general practitioners there is no appreciable difference between 1950 and 1954 or between public and private school graduates in the proportion in partnership practice, except for a tendency for partnerships to be more common among public than private school graduates in 1954; furthermore, there is virtually no change when current and anticipated partnership choices are compared. The anticipated shift away from solo practice is compensated for by a rise in group practice. The proportion of general practitioners in group practice increased from 10 percent to 18 percent (public schools) and from 8 percent to 13 percent (private schools) between the 1950 and 1954 classes, and in all four groupings there is a rise from current to anticipated choice of group practice. In general, group practice is somewhat more favored by public school graduates. Finally, it is noteworthy that hospital practice, both current and anticipated, accounts for only a negligible proportion of general practitioners.

The contention that general practice is the great stronghold of solo practice is confirmed when general practitioners are compared with all other doctors. In both 1950 and 1954, among private school graduates the difference between general practitioners and other doctors choosing solo practice was significant at better than the 5 percent level (CR 2.2 for each year); among public school graduates, the general practitioners' preference for this type of practice was similarly significant (CR 2.5 for each year). There was no significant difference between general practitioners graduating from public and private schools in choice of solo practice.

A similar and very high difference is found between the percentage of general practitioners and of all other doctors in hospital practice, with far fewer general practitioners choosing this type of practice. In the 1954 classes this difference was significant both among private school graduates (CR 5.7) and public school graduates (CR 10.0). In 1950 the difference was significant in public schools (CR 6.2) and also in the private schools (CR 6.4).

Table 8 shows the current status and anticipated choices of internists. Again solo practice is the current choice of a majority in the 1950 class, but a change to other types of practice is anticipated; it is the choice of a smaller proportion in the 1954 class, and further attrition in solo practice is evident in the "anticipated" choices. As was the case with general practitioners, solo practice is more favored (as both a current and anticipated choice) by private than by public school graduates of the 1950 class (CR 2.1), but this difference almost disappears in 1954.

Among internists the anticipated decline in solo practice is compensated for by an increase in group practice and partnership. The proportion currently in group practice shows an absolute rise (among both public and private school graduates) from 1950 to 1954, and there is a similar rise in those planning to be in group or partnership practice at the peaks of their careers. In both years group practice is more favored by public than by private school graduates.

Hospital practice is a much more common status in 1954 than in 1950, again probably reflecting those who are still in training; 11 percent of the private school graduates of 1954 indicated they plan to continue in hospital practice.

TABLE 8. Percentage distribution of internists by present type of practice relationship, 1961, and type anticipated at peak of career, by type of school and year of graduation

| Practice relationship | 1950 Public | | 1950 Private | | 1954 Public | | 1954 Private | |
|---|---|---|---|---|---|---|---|---|
| | Now | Anticipated | Now | Anticipated | Now | Anticipated | Now | Anticipated |
| Solo | 50 | 31 | 69 | 54 | 37 | 29 | 40 | 33 |
| Group | 23 | 27 | 12 | 19 | 27 | 37 | 19 | 26 |
| Hospital | 15 | 8 | 7 | 3 | 24 | 5 | 28 | 11 |
| Partnership | 12 | 25 | 9 | 15 | 8 | 24 | 9 | 13 |
| Other | 0 | 2 | 3 | 0 | 4 | 0 | 4 | 7 |
| No response | 0 | 8 | 0 | 9 | 0 | 4 | 1 | 10 |
| | (52) | | (74) | | (75) | | (105) | |

Table 9 presents similar data for surgeons. Among the 1950 graduates, from both public and private institutions, the largest proportion is currently in solo practice, but a sharp decline is anticipated. The shift will be to group practice and partnership, with the bulk of the increase—particularly among public school graduates—appearing in partnership. Group practice is more favored by public school graduates than by private school graduates of 1950, both currently and in terms of anticipated career plans. Among the 1954 graduates who are now surgeons fewer are in solo practice now, and further attrition may be expected at least among public school graduates because of the anticipated shift to partnership or group practice. The tendency for group practice to be more favored by public school graduates, which was clear in the 1950 class, is not nearly so marked in the 1954 class.

*Present Location of Practice*

In Table 10 the distribution of the doctors in the various specialties is shown in relation to their practice location in 1961. There does not appear to be any definite differences in the distribution of the public and the private medical school graduates, with the exception of those who had located in towns of less than 10,000. Eight and six percent of the private medical school graduates reported that they were practicing in such locations, whereas 14 and 12 percent of the public school graduates in the 1950 and 1954 classes, respectively, reported similar situations. While the public-private school difference here is quite definite (CR 4.5 in 1950, 2.8 in 1954), the small decline from 1950 to 1954 is not. There is no definite change in the distribution of

TABLE 9. Percentage distribution of surgeons by present type of practice relationship, 1961, and type anticipated at peak of career, by type of school and year of graduation

| Practice relationship | 1950 Public | | 1950 Private | | 1954 Public | | 1954 Private | |
|---|---|---|---|---|---|---|---|---|
| | Now | Anticipated | Now | Anticipated | Now | Anticipated | Now | Anticipated |
| Solo | 42 | 24 | 52 | 35 | 28 | 20 | 28 | 29 |
| Group | 28 | 32 | 14 | 18 | 14 | 23 | 10 | 19 |
| Hospital | 10 | 2 | 10 | 5 | 38 | 5 | 41 | 11 |
| Partnership | 18 | 36 | 22 | 33 | 19 | 42 | 11 | 32 |
| Other | 2 | 0 | 1 | 1 | 2 | 3 | 9 | 3 |
| No response | 0 | 6 | 1 | 7 | 0 | 6 | 1 | 6 |
| | (50) | | (94) | | (64) | | (122) | |

TABLE 10. Percentage distribution of doctors by present location of practice, by type of school and year of graduation

| Present location of practice | Public | | Private | |
|---|---|---|---|---|
| | 1950 | 1954 | 1950 | 1954 |
| Town, small town, rural areas (-9,999) | 14 | 12 | 8 | 6 |
| Medium city (10,000-99,999) | 19 | 22 | 22 | 17 |
| Large city (100,000-) | 40 | 39 | 45 | 37 |
| Suburbs[a] | 18 | 11 | 18 | 15 |
| Foreign-military | 5 | 8 | 3 | 9 |
| No response-not applicable | 4 | 7 | 4 | 15 |
| | (334) | (498) | (430) | (509) |

[a]Part of standard Metropolitan Statistical Area, population of segment less than 50,000 and within 20 miles of central city.

doctors in other areas between the 1950 and 1954 classes. The question as to practice location was not applicable to many in the class of 1954 since they were still in training.

About 38 percent of the 1960 United States population lived in areas of under 50,000 population. The fact that only 6 to 14 percent of the physicians in this sample chose to practice in these areas illustrates why rural areas and small cities feel shortages of doctors. The suburbs, which contain about 30 percent of the country's population, attracted only 11 to 18 percent of the graduates of the twelve schools included in this study. Suburbs, by definition, are close to cities, so that this lower rate of recruitment of physicians probably does not have the same significance as the lower rate of recruitment into small cities, towns, and rural areas. Over half of the medical school graduates who participated in this study settled in medium-sized or larger cities (population 50,000 or more) where about one third of the population reside.

The doctor distribution by field of practice and location does not show any characteristic difference between public and private school graduates nor does it vary consistently between 1950 and 1954. Table 11 combines all of the graduates, public and private, 1950 and 1954, to show location of practice by more frequent specialties. The internists, surgeons, and other specialists (pediatricians, obstetricians-gynecologists, pathologists, radiologists, and others) overwhelmingly selected the larger cities as their practice location. Whereas about one third of the population lives in such areas, about two thirds of the specialists practice in them. These specialties are underrepresented in the suburban areas in relation to the proportion of the population living there. However, the small proportion of specialists attracted by the small cities, towns, and rural areas presents the most striking disparity when compared with the population resident in these places.

The general practitioners are the only group that are distributed in appropriate proportion to the population, but, even here, it is evident that they are attracted more frequently by the medium and largest cities than they are by suburban areas or small cities and towns.

TABLE 11. Percentage distribution of all groups by location of present practice by certain fields of practice, 1961

| Location of present practice | Percent of total United States population | General practitioners | Internists | Surgeons | Other |
|---|---|---|---|---|---|
| Medium and large cities (10,000-) | 32 | 40 | 70 | 59 | 67 |
| Town, small town rural area (-9,999) | 38 | 33 | 4 | 5 | 2 |
| Suburb | 30 | 24 | 12 | 11 | 14 |
| No response-not applicable and other | -- | 3 | 14 | 25 | 17 |
| | -- | (381) | (306) | (330) | (754) |

## Hospital Appointments

Virtually all doctors in the sample have hospital appointments (Table 12). A number of doctors were still in training in 1961, as can be seen from the reported hospital appointments either as resident or chief resident. The type of hospital appointment reported did not vary by the doctor's field of practice. General practitioners, for example, reported that they were chief of service with about the same frequency as did doctors in other fields.

TABLE 12. Percentage distribution of doctors by type of hospital appointment, year of graduation, and type of school

| Hospital appointment | 1950 Public | 1950 Private | 1954 Public | 1954 Private |
|---|---|---|---|---|
| Chief of service | 15 | 16 | 8 | 7 |
| Chief resident | 1 | 1 | 2 | 6 |
| Resident | 3 | 0 | 5 | 7 |
| Attending physician | 56 | 58 | 56 | 47 |
| Other | 14 | 17 | 16 | 22 |
| None, no response, not applicable | 12 | 9 | 13 | 11 |
|  | (334) | (430) | (498) | (509) |

## Practice Income

As part of the investigation of the circumstances of their present practice, the doctors were asked several questions about their income. The distribution of all doctors and certain specialties is shown in Table 13 by their reported 1961 net or taxable income from medical practice. The incomes of the public and private medical school graduates were not very different, but there were definite differences between those graduating in 1950 and 1954. Nearly half of the 1950 graduates had net incomes in excess of $20,000 per annum whereas only 28 percent of the public and 14 percent of the private school graduates of 1954 had incomes in this range.

General practitioners achieved a high income sooner than did doctors in other fields. Over half of the general practitioners had incomes of over $20,000 in 1961. This high level apparently was reached quickly, for the 1950 and 1954 graduates reported essentially similar incomes. The internists, whose training postpones the beginning of practice by several years as compared with the general practitioners, had lower incomes. Although the internists who graduated in 1950 had almost caught up with the general practitioners, those who graduated in 1954 had not. The internists who finished medical school in 1954 had, on average, been in practice for three years at the time of the survey. The surgeons, whose training is about the same length as the internists, seem to reach high income levels somewhat more rapidly. One reward of general practice, with its shorter training period, seems to be the acquisition of a high income sooner. This advantage is transitory, however, since physicians who acquire more training (at low incomes) do catch up financially within a few years.

The doctors were also asked to indicate what they anticipated their income would be at the peak of their career. Over 40 percent of the 1950 graduates expected their peak income to be above $30,000 per year. The surgeons were different from all other doctors in that two thirds or more anticipated incomes

TABLE 13. Percentage distribution of doctors by 1961 taxable income, by year of graduation, type of school, and field of practice

|  | Public | | | | Private | | | |
|---|---|---|---|---|---|---|---|---|
|  | All | General practice | Medicine | Surgery | All | General practice | Medicine | Surgery |
| | | | | 1950 | | | | |
| $0-$9,999 | 0 | 5 | 6 | 12 | 11 | 7 | 12 | 10 |
| $10,000-$19,999 | 42 | 40 | 58 | 34 | 42 | 41 | 41 | 34 |
| $20,000 & over | 46 | 53 | 35 | 48 | 44 | 51 | 45 | 55 |
| No response | 3 | 2 | 2 | 6 | 3 | 2 | 3 | 1 |
|  | (334) | (116) | (52) | (50) | (430) | (61) | (74) | (94) |
| | | | | 1954 | | | | |
| $0-$9,999 | 28 | 12 | 41 | 45 | 39 | 10 | 35 | 52 |
| $10,000-$19,999 | 42 | 34 | 49 | 30 | 45 | 33 | 54 | 39 |
| $20,000 & over | 28 | 52 | 8 | 20 | 14 | 58 | 10 | 8 |
| No response | 2 | 2 | 1 | 5 | 2 | 0 | 1 | 2 |
|  | (498) | (164) | (75) | (64) | (509) | (40) | (105) | (122) |

within this range; this is probably a realistic expectation. Among 1954 graduates the surgeons again counted on higher incomes than did doctors in other fields.

The respondents reported medical income from several sources; the major ones were salary and patient fees. Thirty-six and forty-six percent of the 1950 public and private school graduates, respectively, reported salary income. The corresponding percents reported by the 1954 graduates were 55 percent (public) and 70 percent (private).

Table 14 shows the distribution of doctors who reported salary income as a proportion of total income. The private school graduates more frequently reported a high level of salary income than did the public school graduates. The proportion of total income obtained from salary was greater in 1954 than in 1950.

TABLE 14. Percentage distribution of doctors reporting salary income as proportion of total medical income by type of school and year of graduation

| Percentage of income from salary | Public | | Private | |
| --- | --- | --- | --- | --- |
| | 1950 | 1954 | 1950 | 1954 |
| -50% | 79 | 60 | 72 | 45 |
| 51%-100% | 20 | 40 | 28 | 54 |
| No response | 1 | 0 | 0 | 1 |
| | (334) | (498) | (430) | (509) |

The finding that a large proportion of 1950 and 1954 graduates had some salary income cannot be accounted for by men who are still in training. For example, only 4 percent of the 1950 public school graduates and 1 percent of the private school graduates were still in training in 1961. Thirty-six percent and forty-eight percent of the graduates in these two groups reported salary income in that year. The corresponding figures for 1954 show somewhat more men still in residency, but the number is still insufficient to account for the large percentage who reported salary income.

*Value Orientations*

In deciding upon a field of practice and in making decisions about training for practice, a doctor's attitudes and values are deeply involved, consciously or unconsciously. The technical problems presented by this type of questionnaire study did not make extensive exploration of this field feasible. To assess the doctors' values, the following question was asked about how he would judge a fellow physician. "Assuming that a fundamental criterion for identifying a good doctor is his clinical diagnostic ability, how important do you consider each of the following additional criteria to be in identifying a good doctor? (a) His ability to establish rapport with patients. (b) His ability to discern and deal with social and psychological problems of patients. (c) The recognition given him by his colleagues. (d) The research and publications he has to his credit." The doctors' ranking of these criteria was used to group the responses into three categories, strongly patient-oriented, weakly patient-oriented, and professional or mixed orientation.

Overall, about two in three doctors were strongly patient-oriented—that is, in judging a doctor they placed high value on understanding of patients and rapport with patients. There was little difference between public and private school graduates or between the 1950 and 1954 classes in this respect.

There were some fairly consistent differences, however, between doctors in different fields of practice (Table 15). In both the 1950 and 1954 classes general practitioners were strongly patient-oriented; they differed significantly from all other doctors (CR range 2.6 to 6.6) in this respect. Internists, when compared with all other doctors, were not significantly more patient-oriented in 1950 or in 1954, public or private. Psychiatrists from both public and private schools were significantly more strongly patient-oriented than all other doctors in 1954 (CR 3.6 private, 2.4 public) but not in 1950. In contrast, surgeons valued rapport with patients significantly less frequently than all other doctors and tended much more often to have a professional or mixed orientation, giving greater weight to recognition by colleagues (CR range 2.1 to 4.2). In this they resembled doctors engaged in teaching and research.

*Marital Status*

Overall, about 90 percent of the doctors who returned the questionnaire reported that they were married. Five to nine percent in different groups were single and the small remainder were divorced, separated, or widowed. There are some differences in the marital status of doctors who had selected different fields of practice. About 3 percent of general practitioners remained single in all groups in contrast to internists, among whom 8 to 13 percent in the various groups were unmarried. Marriage will receive further attention in later chapters. As will become clear, the time of marriage appears to be an important influence in a doctor's decisions about practice and short training for practice. The general practitioner is quite different from other doctors in this respect.

TABLE 15. Percentage distribution of doctors by value orientation and by field of practice, type of school and year of graduation

| | 1950 | | | | | 1954 | | | | |
|---|---|---|---|---|---|---|---|---|---|---|
| | General practice | Medicine | Surgery | Psychiatry | Teaching/ research | General practice | Medicine | Surgery | Psychiatry | Teaching/ research |
| **Public** | | | | | | | | | | |
| Strong patient | 78 | 60 | 40 | 67 | 42 | 73 | 56 | 61 | 82 | 47 |
| Weak patient | 10 | 8 | 18 | 13 | 21 | 12 | 16 | 9 | 9 | 16 |
| Professional or mixed | 12 | 31 | 38 | 17 | 32 | 14 | 25 | 27 | 6 | 34 |
| No response | 0 | 2 | 4 | 4 | 5 | 1 | 3 | 3 | 3 | 3 |
| | (116) | (52) | (50) | (24) | (19) | (164) | (75) | (64) | (33) | (38) |
| **Private** | | | | | | | | | | |
| Strong patient | 74 | 70 | 52 | 70 | 58 | 65 | 53 | 55 | 80 | 51 |
| Weak patient | 10 | 11 | 14 | 12 | 12 | 13 | 27 | 9 | 6 | 15 |
| Professional or mixed | 16 | 16 | 33 | 15 | 29 | 23 | 18 | 34 | 14 | 33 |
| No response | 0 | 3 | 1 | 3 | 2 | 0 | 0 | 2 | 0 | 1 |
| | (61) | (74) | (94) | (33) | (59) | (40) | (105) | (122) | (35) | (86) |

# IV / Decisions about a Field of Practice

WHAT LEADS DOCTORS to choose one field of practice in preference to another? Obviously their personal interests are important, but these personal interests in turn have multiple roots. The interests of a doctor who has grown up in a small town and whose father was the town doctor will probably differ greatly from the interests of a doctor who was raised in or near a large, bustling industrial metropolis and whose father worked on the assembly line of a factory. The doctor whose several brothers have all gone into business will quite likely differ in his interests from the one who is the only child of a college professor.

The doctor's social and economic circumstances while he was a student in medical school may also affect decisions about the professional career he chooses. Working and associating for four years with other students may shape the student's interest and influence the direction he takes after graduation. Furthermore, financial resources and family obligations are likely to encourage or circumscribe the student's plans for a career. In comparison with a student who has no family or financial obligations, a married student with several children and limited financial resources may need a much stronger inducement to choose a field of practice that demands a long residency. The perceived characteristics of different fields of practice and the prestige and income associated with them may also influence choice. A variety of social, economic, and cultural circumstances must be considered in assessing why particular career decisions were made. William Schofield, writing in Gee and Glazer's *The Ecology of the Medical Student*(11), has suggested that these circumstances may be

# DECISIONS ABOUT FIELD OF PRACTICE

summarized as: (1) family traditions and pressures; (2) social prestige attached to the profession; (3) promise of economic return; (4) social demand for practitioners; (5) development of a strong identification with another individual who is in the given line of work; (6) an unusual opportunity or encouragement early in life; (7) an unusual restriction or handicap which fastens interest on the profession associated with its study (polio, tuberculosis, and so forth); (8) personal interests, values.

Although each of these circumstances could not be analyzed in detail for the 1771 respondents in this study, an attempt was made to ascertain the relationship between the respondents' choices of specialty or general practice and some of the major social, economic, and cultural factors associated with their backgrounds and circumstances in medical school.

## Influences Reported by Doctors on Field of Practice Decisions

The respondents were asked to what extent their decision about a field of practice was influenced by intellectual interests; feeling of identity with certain types of patients (children, aged); financial circumstances; social circumstances (marriage plans, influence of friends, postponed social plans, and so forth); or spouse's expectations or needs. The largest proportion of the respondents (from 72 percent to 87 percent in the various groups) indicated that intellectual interests had been a major influence on this decision (Table 16). About one third of the respondents reported being influenced by their interest in certain types of patients, and one tenth to a quarter indicated that financial circumstances were important. Social pressures and spouse's expectations and needs were less frequently mentioned.

TABLE 16. Percent of doctors strongly influenced in choice of a field of practice by factor, all doctors, by field of practice, year of graduation, and type of school

| Influential factor | All doctors | | General practitioners | | Medicine | | Surgery | | Teaching and research | |
|---|---|---|---|---|---|---|---|---|---|---|
| | 1950 | 1954 | 1950 | 1954 | 1950 | 1954 | 1950 | 1954 | 1950 | 1954 |
| | | | | | Public | | | | | |
| Intellectual interests | 72 | 74 | 54 | 54 | 96 | 92 | 72 | 83 | 84 | 92 |
| Patient interests | 34 | 36 | 48 | 48 | 19 | 21 | 14 | 16 | 21 | 21 |
| Finances | 29 | 22 | 56 | 45 | 8 | 4 | 20 | 20 | -- | 8 |
| Social pressures | 21 | 15 | 35 | 24 | 8 | 4 | 16 | 8 | 5 | 8 |
| Spouse's expectations and needs | 18 | 11 | 35 | 20 | 12 | 1 | 4 | 5 | 5 | 3 |
| Other | 17 | 19 | -- | -- | -- | -- | -- | -- | -- | -- |
| | (334) | (498) | (116) | (164) | (52) | (75) | (50) | (64) | (19) | (38) |
| | | | | | Private | | | | | |
| Intellectual interests | 81 | 87 | 59 | 60 | 92 | 93 | 83 | 90 | 97 | 100 |
| Patient interests | 31 | 27 | 49 | 40 | 18 | 20 | 15 | 18 | 17 | 19 |
| Finances | 18 | 11 | 48 | 43 | 9 | 9 | 15 | 10 | 10 | 7 |
| Social pressures | 12 | 10 | 33 | 33 | 7 | 8 | 8 | 8 | 8 | 3 |
| Spouse's expectations and needs | 10 | 9 | 25 | 28 | 8 | 8 | 7 | 6 | 8 | 5 |
| Other | 17 | 15 | -- | -- | -- | -- | -- | -- | -- | -- |
| | (430) | (509) | (61) | (40) | (74) | (105) | (94) | (122) | (59) | (86) |

Intellectual interests were stated to be important more often by the private school respondents than by those from the public schools. While 81 percent and 87 percent of private school graduates in 1950 and 1954 said they were much influenced by this factor, only 72 percent and 74 percent of the public school graduates of these years responded similarly. This difference is not significant for 1950, but is for 1954 (CR 1.7 and 3.5).

Interest in certain types of patients and financial circumstances were more important in the public than the private school groups. This was especially true of financial circumstances —29 percent and 23 percent of the 1950 and 1954 public school respondents stated that finances were important, as compared with 18 percent and 11 percent of the 1950 and 1954 private school respondents, and these differences are significant (CR 2.4 and 3.5).

If doctors are grouped according to the field of practice they reported in 1961, it is apparent that quite different combinations of factors influenced the choices of each group.

*General practice.* Doctors who had chosen general practice were less influenced than all other respondents by intellectual interests, and more influenced by their interest in patients, financial circumstances, social pressures, and spouses' expectations and needs; these differences are significant. Only 57 to 60 percent of the general practitioners indicated that intellectual interests were important, compared to 84 to 90 percent of all other respondents; this difference is significant, both in public and private schools, in both 1950 and 1954 (CR 4.9 and 7.3 in public schools, 4.1 and 4.1 in private schools, in 1950 and 1954). Conversely, general practitioners listed financial circumstances as important influences on field-of-practice choice much more often than did other doctors; in 1950, 59 percent of the public school and 52 percent of the private school general practitioners reported this influence, as compared to only 17 percent of all other public school graduates and 15 percent of all other private school graduates (CR for difference is 6.9 for public school graduates, 4.0 for private school graduates). The greater importance to general practitioners of financial circumstances was equally significant in 1954 (CR 5.5 in public schools, 6.7 in private schools).

Similarly, interest in certain types of patients was reported to be an important influence significantly more often by general practitioners than other respondents in both public and private schools in 1950 (CR 4.3 and 4.2) and in public schools in 1954 (CR 4.1), with more than half the general practitioners listing this factor as compared to less than a third of all other doctors.

The percentage of general practitioners reporting social pressures as an important influence on career choice ranged from 25 to 37, while only 8 to 14 percent of all other doctors listed social pressures (CR 5.0 and 3.9 in public schools, 2.6 and 3.4 in private schools, 1950 and 1954).

Finally, general practitioners were significantly more likely to list spouse's expectations or needs as an important influence. In 1950, 41 percent of the public school general practitioners did so (versus only 12 percent of all other public school graduates) and 31 percent of private school general practitioners did so (versus only 11 percent of all other private school graduates); similar differences between general practitioners and all other doctors were found in 1954 (CR 5.9 and 5.1 in public schools, 1.9 and 2.5 in private schools, 1950 and 1954).

In summary, then, general practitioners were significantly different from all other doctors in the reported influences on their choice of a field of practice—more influenced by finances, social pressures, their spouses, and interest in certain types of patients, and less influenced by intellectual interests. These characteristics overrode any differences between public and private school graduates: among all general practitioners no significant difference between public and private school graduates was found.

*Internal medicine.* Intellectual interest had a greater influence on internists' choice of specialty than on the choices of any other group of respondents with the single exception of teachers and research workers. From 92 to 98 percent of internists in public and private schools, and in both 1950 and 1954, indicated they were influenced by this factor. In comparison, this influence was reported by 72 to 87 percent of all other doctors; the difference between internists and others was significant (CR range 4.1 to 6.0) except among private school graduates in 1954. Its importance is further highlighted by the fact that fewer internists (as compared to all other doctors) indicated they were influenced by special interest in patients, financial circumstances, social pressures, or spouses' expectations.

*Surgery.* The percent of surgeons influenced by intellectual interests in the choice of their specialty was about the same as that for all respondents in the study. As compared with all other doctors, however, significantly fewer surgeons were influenced by special interest in patients. Only 16 to 20 percent reported this influence, compared to 30 to 42 percent of nonsurgeons (CR 4.6 and 5.7 in public schools, 3.9 and 2.2 in private schools, 1950 and 1954). No marked differences between surgeons and nonsurgeons appeared with regard to financial circumstances, social pressures, or spouse's expectations.

*Teaching and research.* The graduates who were teachers and research workers overwhelmingly reported that they were influenced by intellectual interests in selecting their careers. In the private schools nearly 100 percent so reported; the corresponding proportions in the public schools were 84 percent of the 1950 and 92 percent of the 1954 classes.

This emphasis on intellectual interests was especially marked when teachers and researchers were compared with all other doctors (CR 2.1 and 5.0 in public schools, and 6.5 and 4.5 in private schools, 1950 and 1954).

Financial circumstances, social pressures, and spouse's expectations were of little importance in making the decision to follow a teaching or research career. Less than 10 percent of teacher-researchers indicated they were much influenced by any of these considerations.

*Other specialties.* The pediatricians were the only group in which intellectual interests were not the most frequently reported consideration in choice of a career. Except among the 1954 public school graduates, interest in certain types of patients was reported to be important more frequently than intellectual interests. When pediatricians were compared with all other physicians, this emphasis on interest in patients was significant (CR 8.6 and 6.1 in public schools, and 6.9 and 12.0 in private schools, 1950 and 1954).

In general, the responses of obstetrician-gynecologists were similar to those of pediatricians, especially in interest in patients. As compared with all other physicians, obstetrician-gynecologists from the private schools (but not the public schools) in both 1950 and 1954 reported patient interest significantly more frequently as an important influence on career choice.

## *Father's Background and Education*

The education of the father of a medical student might have both direct or indirect effects upon the student's career and subsequent choice of a field of practice. It is known that education and income are related, with larger incomes being associated with more education. Thus, the influence of education might really be an indirect one relating to family finances. A substantial number of medical students (approximately one in eight in the present study) have fathers who are doctors; as we will see later, these students are among those with the longest residency training. Either finances or family educational tradition might explain this.

About half of the doctors reported that their fathers had obtained a high school education or less (Table 17). About a fourth of the doctors had fathers who had gone to college or graduated from college, and another fourth had fathers with postgraduate college educations, including, of course, the fathers who were doctors. There was only one significant difference between the public and private school graduates' descriptions of their fathers' education; in 1954 more fathers of the private school graduates had done postgraduate work (CR 2.6).

The data presented in Table 15 suggested that teachers and researchers, in general, had fathers with more education, and that general practitioners, as a rule, had fathers with less education than was the case with other physicians. To examine this possibility more clearly, the data were regrouped to permit comparison of teachers and researchers with all others and of general practitioners with all others, with respect to father's education. These comparisons yielded rather few significant findings. Among general practitioners, for example, significantly fewer 1954 graduates of the public schools had fathers with postgraduate educations. Among teachers and researchers the tendency to have fewer fathers with no college training was significant in one class (private schools, 1950), as was the higher proportion of fathers with postgraduate training (public schools, 1954).

TABLE 17. Percentage distribution of doctors by father's education, field of practice, type of school, and year of graduation

| Years of father's college education | 1950 | | | | 1954 | | | |
|---|---|---|---|---|---|---|---|---|
| | All doctors | General practice | Teaching and research | All others | All doctors | General practice | Teaching and research | All others |
| | | | | Public | | | | |
| None | 53 | 55 | 43 | 53 | 53 | 60 | 42 | 51 |
| 1-4 years | 21 | 22 | 37 | 19 | 25 | 24 | 18 | 26 |
| More than 4 years | 23 | 19 | 21 | 24 | 20 | 14 | 39 | 22 |
| No response | 3 | 3 | 0 | 3 | 1 | 1 | 0 | 1 |
| | (334) | (116) | (19) | (199) | (498) | (164) | (38) | (296) |
| | | | | Private | | | | |
| None | 50 | 61 | 37 | 49 | 42 | 58 | 36 | 42 |
| 1-4 years | 22 | 18 | 36 | 21 | 25 | 20 | 28 | 25 |
| More than 4 years | 26 | 20 | 27 | 28 | 32 | 23 | 34 | 32 |
| No response | 2 | 2 | 0 | 2 | 1 | 0 | 2 | 0 |
| | (430) | (61) | (59) | (310) | (509) | (40) | (86) | (383) |

Medical students are a highly selected group.(1, 5) One of the many ways in which this is apparent is shown in Table 18, in which the occupations of the fathers of the graduates of these six private and six public medical schools are compared with the occupational distribution of the United States population. The most striking example of selection is furnished by the doctors

TABLE 18. Percentage distribution of employed persons, U.S., 1950, by occupation and occupations of fathers of 1950 and 1954 medical school graduates

| Occupational group | United States[a] total | Doctors' fathers |
|---|---|---|
| Physicians | 0.4 | 13.0 |
| Professional | 4.4 | 17.6 |
| Executive | 4.9 | 9.9 |
| Small business | 5.4 | 19.5 |
| Semi-professional/ clerical | 15.6 | 14.8 |
| Crafts[b] | 57.6 | 17.7 |
| Other[c] | 10.3 | 5.8 |
| No response | 1.1 | 1.6 |
|  |  | (1771) |

[a]Statistical Abstracts of the United States, 1960, Department of Commerce, U.S. Bureau of Census, p. 218.

[b]Includes skilled and unskilled laborers.

[c]Includes farmers. In "Doctors' fathers" column it includes a few sons of military men.

whose fathers were also doctors. Although physicians represent less than one half of one percent of the United States employed population, 13 percent of all medical students reported this background. There was also a strong selection from other professional groups as well as from among those classified as executives. And fathers who were small businessmen were overrepresented in the group of doctors studied. The small business, executive, and professional group (including physicians), which constitutes approximately 15 percent of the employed United States population, contributed about 60 percent of all medical students. Fathers who were in semiprofessional and clerical occupations were represented in about the same proportion as their percentage of the total population, whereas the crafts (which includes all blue collar workers) were markedly underrepresented.

The family backgrounds of British medical students is interesting in this connection. While the British occupational classification is not precisely the same as the American, it is sufficiently similar to suggest that the selection of British medical students is very much like that in the United States. About 50 percent of the British medical students reported managerial or professional backgrounds, indicating that in England, as in the United States, medical school students are selected mainly from a rather small segment of the population.(3)

There is some suggestion that the fields of practice reported by the doctors in this study vary in relation to their father's occupations. Thirty-seven and 36 percent of all the public school graduates in 1950 and 1954, respectively, reported that their fathers were physicians, executives, or professional men; of the public school general practitioners 37 and 27 percent (in the same years) had fathers in this group. The figures for all private school graduates who reported fathers with physician, executive,

## DECISIONS ABOUT FIELD OF PRACTICE 59

or professional occupations were 39 and 48 percent in 1950 and 1954; the general practitioner graduates of the private schools reported fathers in these categories in 31 and 41 percent of instances in 1950 and 1954.

Doctors who are now in teaching or research positions were somewhat different from all doctors with regard to their fathers' occupations: 53 and 55 percent of their fathers were professional men or executives in the case of the public school graduates, and 47 and 53 percent in the case of the private school graduates in 1950 and 1954 respectively. When teachers and researchers were compared with all others in this respect, however, only one significant difference appeared: among public school graduates in 1954, the fathers of teachers and researchers more frequently were in the physician-executive-professional category (CR 2.4).

The ethnic origin of doctors' fathers seems to have little influence upon a doctor's selection of a field of practice with a single curious exception. Doctors who reported that their fathers were born in Eastern Europe and the Eastern Mediterranean area (that is, the Balkans and the Near East) entered general practice at a much lower rate than did those whose fathers were born elsewhere, including other parts of Europe or the United States. This difference was significant among public but not private school graduates in both 1950 and 1954 (CR 3.4 and 3.2). This small group of doctors tended to be overrepresented in the practice of internal medicine, although this reached significance only among public school graduates in 1950 (CR 4.1). The finding was not related to religious preference. The group of doctors whose fathers were born in Eastern Europe and the Eastern Mediterranean were also different from all doctors with respect to their hospital training, as will be discussed in the next chapter.

The age of the father of a medical student might have some influence upon a doctor's career in medical school. Different ages are accompanied by different levels of earnings; the aid that a student could anticipate from his family would probably vary markedly if his father were in a period of high earnings in middle life or approaching the reduced income of retirement.

General practitioners reported older fathers than did all other doctors. This was not marked for the class of 1950; however, when general practitioners of the class of 1954 were compared with all other doctors in relation to the proportion with fathers aged sixty-three or more at the time of the respondent's entry into medical school, a significantly higher proportion was found among general practitioners in the public schools (CR 2.5).

*Family Composition*

The number of brothers and sisters that a medical student has and their age relationship to him might be expected to influence his decisions about training and practice. A larger number of siblings might curtail a family's ability to support a doctor through extensive training, whereas an older brother or sister who was employed might be a source of support. Younger brothers or sisters might act as a greater constraint upon the doctor's education and training than older siblings. However, the examination of the family composition of the doctors at the time they were in medical school revealed rather little, except perhaps to indicate in a second way the extent to which medicine is a "family" profession.

Thus, among the doctors who reported that they had older brothers employed, approximately 10 percent in all groups reported that they had a brother who was a doctor. It will be

## DECISIONS ABOUT FIELD OF PRACTICE

recalled that 13 percent of respondents reported that their fathers were doctors. The respondents in this study who had physician brothers were more frequently surgeons than in any other type of practice; why this should be so is not evident from the data. General practitioners' brothers were more often craftsmen and laborers than was true for the brothers of specialists. Contrariwise, the general practitioners had fewer brothers engaged in executive occupations. There were no marked differences in brothers' occupations for the other specialists.

*Geographic Distribution*

Medical students appear to be selected differentially from different parts of the United States population. In 1930 less than half of the United States population lived in standard metropolitan areas. Yet, two thirds or more of the doctors who participated in this study were born in these areas. Even within these classifications there is further evidence of selection. Approximately one third of the United States population in 1930 lived in the central cities within standard metropolitan areas, whereas well over half of the doctors reported that they were born in the central city (Table 19).

The selection of a medical school and the choice of some fields of practice seem to be related to the doctor's place of birth, as is illustrated in Table 19. The public school graduates were drawn more frequently from the areas classified here as small city, town, or rural area. The private school graduates were drawn less frequently from this part of the population and to a greater extent from the large city.

The general practitioners—both public and private school graduates—more frequently reported birth in a small city, town,

TABLE 19. Percentage distribution of doctors by place of birth for all doctors and certain specialties, 1950 and 1954 graduates combined

| Place of birth | Percent of total U.S. population 1930 | All doctors | | General practitioners | | Psychiatrists | | Teaching and research | |
|---|---|---|---|---|---|---|---|---|---|
| | | Public | Private | Public | Private | Public | Private | Public | Private |
| Central and large cities 50,000 or greater | 35 | 59 | 70 | 51 | 51 | 67 | 76 | 75 | 70 |
| Small city, town, rural area under 50,000 | 46 | 31 | 17 | 41 | 35 | 25 | 13 | 14 | 10 |
| Suburb | 19 | 6 | 6 | 5 | 8 | 7 | 9 | 7 | 8 |
| No response and other | -- | 4 | 6 | 3 | 6 | 2 | 1 | 2 | 12 |
| | | (832) | (939) | (280) | (101) | (57) | (68) | (57) | (145) |

or rural area, though this was significant only in the 1954 class. A correspondingly smaller proportion of the general practitioners were born in large cities. The opposite was true of psychiatrists—but only for those who graduated from private schools (CR 2.9 and 2.1 in 1950 and 1954). Doctors who were in teaching and research in 1961 showed a distribution very similar to that of the psychiatrists. No consistent differences were noted for doctors in other fields of practice.

It is well known that public medical schools tend to select students from within their own geographic area. Presumably, the absence of any such restraint upon the private schools results in a somewhat wider geographic representation within their student bodies.

About two thirds of all the doctors who participated in this study were born in the regions of the United States in which the medical school they attended was located. A variable number, from 3 to 6 percent of the students in the various groups were foreign born. Eighty-one percent of the doctors who graduated from public schools in 1950 reported that they were born in the same region as their medical school; this increased to 83 percent in 1954. A similar trend was seen in the private schools, where 64 percent of the students were born in the region of the school in 1950, increasing to 70 percent in 1954.

*Doctors' Age at Graduation from Medical School*

The age at graduation from medical school is likely to be influenced by many things. Among the 1950 graduates, most of whom entered school in 1946, military service during World War II was an important determinant. Under more usual circumstances a doctor's age at graduation might be determined by his academic ability or by his economic circumstances.

The distribution of doctors by their age at graduation is shown in Table 20. In the class of 1950 the proportion aged twenty-nine or more was significantly greater than in the class of 1954, in both public (CR 4.6) and private (CR 6.2) schools. This undoubtedly reflects the large number of returning veterans who entered medical school in 1946. The private school graduates tended to be younger than the public school graduates in both 1950 and 1954. This difference was not significant for the 1950 graduates, but was for the 1954 groups (CR 2.9).

When age at graduation is examined in comparison with the fields of practice which the doctors reported in 1961, one group —the general practitioners—stands out as quite different from all others. As shown in Table 20, substantially more of them are in the oldest age group and fewer in the youngest group. When the proportion of general practitioners aged twenty-nine or more at graduation is compared with the proportion among all other doctors, the difference is significant (CR 2.0 and 4.0 in public schools, 3.3 and 2.0 in private schools, 1950 and 1954 respectively); there was no public-private difference among general practitioners in this respect. Conversely, the proportion of general practitioners aged less than twenty-four at graduation, compared with others, reached significance only among private school graduates in 1950 (CR 4.3).

While there was a tendency for teachers and researchers to be drawn less frequently from the highest age group and more often from the youngest, this was significant only among private school graduates in 1950.

A high proportion of the public school graduates go into general practice; since the public school general practitioners are, as

TABLE 20. Percentage distribution of doctors by age at graduation, all doctors, general practitioners, teaching/research, by type of school and year of graduation

| Age at graduation | 1950 | | | 1954 | | |
|---|---|---|---|---|---|---|
| | All doctors | General practice | Teaching/research | All doctors | General practice | Teaching/research |
| | | | Public | | | |
| 29- | 47 | 58 | 42 | 22 | 33 | 16 |
| 25-28 | 36 | 33 | 32 | 70 | 62 | 55 |
| -24 | 17 | 9 | 26 | 7 | 5 | 24 |
| No response | 1 | 0 | 0 | 1 | 1 | 5 |
| | (334) | (116) | (19) | (498) | (164) | (38) |
| | | | Private | | | |
| 29- | 37 | 54 | 22 | 11 | 25 | 8 |
| 25-28 | 41 | 38 | 49 | 75 | 68 | 78 |
| -24 | 19 | 3 | 27 | 12 | 3 | 12 |
| No response | 3 | 5 | 2 | 2 | 5 | 2 |
| | (430) | (61) | (59) | (509) | (40) | (86) |

we have seen, older than their classmates, we would expect the remaining public school graduates—the specialists—to be, on the whole, younger than all doctors. This is, indeed, the case. Among the private schools the general practitioners, while older, constitute a small proportion of all graduates, so the specialist group, on the whole, is not different in age from all doctors.

*Economic Circumstances in Medical School*

Although many medical students have families that can be assumed to have comfortable or large incomes, there is a substantial proportion whose family descriptions suggest modest means. Soutter's studies of Boston University students shows that some medical students live on incomes that are within the range of poverty as defined for persons or families qualifying for public welfare in the same area. (28) In an attempt to determine how financial support affected a doctor's education, training, and practice, several questions were asked. The first asked the doctor for the proportion of his total educational costs borne by himself, parents, his spouse, loans, scholarships, as well as other sources of support. Two other questions asked for information on the doctor's yearly earnings while in medical school and the amount of his debt at graduation.

The evidence shows that medical students, in most instances, received support from many sources. Table 21 shows the percentages of doctors who reported a major source of support, defined as more than 50 percent from a single source. About two thirds of all doctors reported a major single source, and this is very similar in 1950 and 1954 in both private and public medical schools.

TABLE 21. Percent of doctors reporting a major source of financial support (>50%) for medical education by source for all doctors by field of practice, type of school, and year of graduation

| Source of support | 1950 | | | | 1954 | | | |
|---|---|---|---|---|---|---|---|---|
| | All doctors | General practice | Medicine | Surgery | All doctors | General practice | Medicine | Surgery |
| *Public* | | | | | | | | |
| Parents | 20 | 11 | 25 | 28 | 32 | 16 | 40 | 36 |
| G.I. bill | 26 | 31 | 21 | 20 | 7 | 12 | 4 | 9 |
| Self | 12 | 12 | 10 | 18 | 14 | 18 | 16 | 13 |
| Spouse | 5 | 6 | 6 | 6 | 7 | 9 | 4 | 3 |
| Loans | 1 | 2 | 0 | 0 | 1 | 1 | 3 | 2 |
| Scholarship | 2 | 2 | 4 | 2 | 1 | 1 | 0 | 0 |
| Other | 1 | 0 | 0 | 0 | 2 | 2 | 1 | 3 |
| | (334) | (116) | (52) | (50) | (498) | (164) | (75) | (64) |
| *Private* | | | | | | | | |
| Parents | 29 | 16 | 23 | 37 | 51 | 25 | 51 | 56 |
| G.I. bill | 22 | 26 | 28 | 22 | 2 | 5 | 1 | 2 |
| Self | 5 | 8 | 4 | 6 | 5 | 8 | 4 | 5 |
| Spouse | 5 | 12 | 3 | 4 | 4 | 8 | 5 | 3 |
| Loans | 1 | 0 | 1 | 1 | 3 | 0 | 3 | 2 |
| Scholarship | 1 | 0 | 1 | 1 | 1 | 0 | 0 | 0 |
| Other | 3 | 2 | 1 | 2 | 3 | 5 | 5 | 2 |
| | (430) | (61) | (74) | (94) | (509) | (40) | (105) | (122) |

The G.I. Education Bill was the most frequent source of major support in 1950, whereas parents were the most frequent source among the 1954 graduates. The proportion of physicians who reported support by parents was higher in the private schools than the public and was higher in 1954 classes of both types of schools than in 1950. The public-private difference in reported frequency of parental support was significant in both 1950 and 1954 (CR 3.1 for 1950 and 4.0 for 1954). The medical students' own earnings were substantially more frequent in the public schools than in the private. The frequency of major self-support was significantly different for both 1950 and 1954 graduates (CR 3.0 for 1950 and 3.8 for 1954). Other sources of major support were uncommon except for spouses' earnings which were reported by 4 to 7 percent of the physicians. For the private school graduate this was about as frequent as self-support.

When major sources of support in medical school are examined with reference to the field of practice reported by the doctor in 1961, it is apparent that there are some associations (Table 21). The 1950 graduates of both the public and the private medical schools who entered general practice listed the G.I. Bill more frequently than any other category as their major source of support. Although the G.I. Bill had declined markedly in importance as a source of support for the 1954 graduates, the general practitioners were still supported more frequently from this source than were all doctors. Although these differences were consistent they were not large or technically significant. The modest differences between the general practitioner graduates of public and private schools did not reach significant levels in either year.

The general practitioners were different from internists and surgeons in another important respect. In both 1950 and 1954, in

DECISIONS ABOUT FIELD OF PRACTICE 69

private and public medical schools, they reported markedly less frequent parental support than did either internists or surgeons —or all doctors. Although the general practitioner graduates of public and private schools reported somewhat different levels of parental support, these differences are neither large nor significant. The differences between the general practitioners and all other doctors were significant, however, within the public (CR 2.5 for 1950 and 2.8 for 1954) and private (CR 2.2 for 1950 and 2.5 for 1954) school groups.

Table 22 shows the minor sources of financial support. This is defined as less than 50 percent of total educational costs. The doctor's own earnings were the most frequent source of minor support. This was more important in 1954 than in 1950. The critical ratio for the 1950–1954 difference for public school graduates was 2.9 and for the private groups, 2.6.

The G.I. Education Bill had declined in importance by 1954 but was still a frequent source of minor support. It was also an important source of minor support in 1950, indicating that in that year a substantial proportion of all medical students received some benefits from this legislation. When these minor sources of support are examined in relation to the doctor's present field of practice, rather few associations are found. The men who were in general practice in 1961 reported that their wives had been a minor source of support with greater frequency than did either the internists or the surgeons. As will be seen later, general practitioners were more frequently married as medical students than any other types of doctors.

Scholarships seldom provide major support but are more important as a minor source. The frequency of scholarships increased sharply between 1950 and 1954. Four percent of the public school graduates of 1950 reported scholarship aid; this

TABLE 22. Percent of doctors reporting minor sources of financial support for medical education (<50%) by source, field of practice, type of school, and year of graduation

| | 1950 | | | | 1954 | | | |
|---|---|---|---|---|---|---|---|---|
| | All doctors | General practice | Medicine | Surgery | All doctors | General practice | Medicine | Surgery |
| | | | | Public | | | | |
| G.I. bill | 35 | 41 | 37 | 24 | 27 | 38 | 19 | 22 |
| Self | 59 | 75 | 65 | 38 | 70 | 70 | 59 | 72 |
| Parents | 26 | 23 | 23 | 40 | 34 | 34 | 39 | 38 |
| Spouse | 25 | 34 | 14 | 18 | 30 | 31 | 31 | 25 |
| Loans | 18 | 24 | 17 | 14 | 24 | 30 | 20 | 22 |
| Scholarships | 4 | 3 | 4 | 4 | 14 | 11 | 13 | 14 |
| | (334) | (116) | (52) | (50) | (498) | (164) | (75) | (64) |
| | | | | Private | | | | |
| G.I. bill | 36 | 41 | 31 | 39 | 19 | 38 | 22 | 16 |
| Self | 56 | 54 | 62 | 57 | 69 | 68 | 70 | 72 |
| Parents | 29 | 21 | 31 | 34 | 31 | 40 | 32 | 29 |
| Spouse | 21 | 31 | 19 | 17 | 20 | 45 | 15 | 16 |
| Loans | 13 | 10 | 19 | 9 | 22 | 33 | 22 | 22 |
| Scholarships | 16 | 7 | 18 | 15 | 23 | 28 | 26 | 18 |
| | (430) | (61) | (74) | (94) | (509) | (40) | (105) | (122) |

percentage increased to 14 among the 1954 classes. The level of scholarship aid reported by private school respondents was somewhat higher, 16 and 23 percent for 1950 and 1954, respectively. These public-private differences were significant in 1950 (CR 2.2) but not in 1954.

Public school graduates reported higher earnings while in medical school than did private school graduates, as is shown in Table 23. Approximately one third of the public school graduates reported that they had earned over $1500 per year while attending medical school, whereas about a quarter of the private school graduates reported earnings at this level. The different proportions of public and private school graduates was at the borderline of significance (CR 1.98) for the 1950 groups and definite in 1954 (CR 2.3). The percent of private school graduates who reported minimal earnings—less than $500 per year—was significantly less than that reported by public school graduates in both 1950 (CR 3.1) and 1954 (CR 2.3).

TABLE 23. Percentage distribution of doctors by yearly earnings while in medical school, all doctors and general practitioners, by type of school and year of graduation

| Yearly earnings | All doctors | | | | General practitioners | | | |
|---|---|---|---|---|---|---|---|---|
| | Public | | Private | | Public | | Private | |
| | 1950 | 1954 | 1950 | 1954 | 1950 | 1954 | 1950 | 1954 |
| 0 - $499 | 31 | 27 | 48 | 42 | 20 | 21 | 39 | 30 |
| $500 - $1499 | 34 | 39 | 26 | 36 | 36 | 38 | 21 | 25 |
| $1500 - | 34 | 34 | 25 | 22 | 42 | 41 | 39 | 45 |
| No response | 2 | 1 | 2 | 0 | 2 | 0 | 0 | 0 |
| | (334) | (498) | (430) | (509) | (116) | (164) | (61) | (40) |

For the most part, general practitioners reported higher earnings in medical school. As can be seen in Table 24, over 40 percent of public school graduates in general practice reported earnings of over $1500 yearly, whereas the corresponding percentages for the private school graduates were 39 and 45 percent in 1950 and 1954 respectively. The differences here are not significant for public school graduates in 1954, but are significant for public school graduates of 1950 (CR 2.1) and for private school graduates of 1950 (CR 2.2) and 1954 (CR 3.0).

TABLE 24. Percentage distribution of doctors by debt at graduation, type of school, and year of graduation

| Debt at graduation | Public | | Private | |
|---|---|---|---|---|
| | 1950 | 1954 | 1950 | 1954 |
| Less than $100 | 65 | 58 | 69 | 63 |
| $101 - $3000 | 23 | 24 | 15 | 22 |
| $3001 - | 11 | 16 | 14 | 15 |
| No Response | 1 | 2 | 2 | 1 |
| | (334) | (498) | (430) | (509) |

The majority of students in both the public and private schools incurred debts of less than $100 by the time of graduation, as is shown in Table 24. Debts of less than $100 would presumably be equivalent to being debt-free, insofar as any limiting effect upon subsequent planning is concerned. In both the public and private schools there were somewhat fewer students in 1954 than in 1950 who reported minimum debt. This was

## DECISIONS ABOUT FIELD OF PRACTICE

significant only for the private school graduates. There was also a corresponding increase from 1950 to 1954 in the number that reported larger debts. A very probable explanation for this is the greater number of students supported by the G.I. Education Bill in 1950. However, this increased frequency of large debts was significant only among the public school graduates (CR 2.4). The data may further suggest that public school graduates were harder hit financially by the decline of the G.I. Bill as a support source. The fact of debt did not seem to be strongly associated with selection of any particular field of practice. General practitioners among both public and private school graduates tended to be underrepresented in the group with no debt and overrepresented in the high-debt group. The trend was quite definite among 1954 graduates but was much less clear in 1950. Although these data suggest that general practitioners finish medical school with more debt than other doctors, the pattern is not sufficiently consistent to demonstrate the case.

When educational debt is examined in relation to father's occupation (see Table 25), it is found that debt is less frequent among sons of doctors, executives, and small businessmen—occupations associated with high incomes. Sons of semiprofessional or clerical workers, craftsmen, and professional men—other than doctors—are more frequently in debt. These are occupations with lower mean incomes. The difference between the essentially debt-free status of the doctors whose fathers followed an occupation with a high average income were consistently and significantly different from the second group whose fathers were members of callings with low average income (CR range, 3.4 to 9.1). Large debt at graduation, defined as over $3,000, was also significantly different in most groups. The frequency of large

TABLE 25. Percent of doctors debt-free at conclusion of medical education by father's occupation

| | | | | Occupation of father | | | |
|---|---|---|---|---|---|---|---|
| | All doctors | Executive | Physician | Small business | Clerical semi-professional | Craftsmen | Professional |
| Public 1950 | 65 (334) | 72 (25) | 70 (37) | 79 (67) | 49 (53) | 61 (56) | 60 (63) |
| Public 1954 | 58 (498) | 84 (44) | 76 (50) | 64 (113) | 53 (66) | 47 (97) | 55 (86) |
| Private 1950 | 69 (430) | 73 (40) | 75 (60) | 82 (87) | 64 (69) | 62 (76) | 58 (69) |
| Private 1954 | 63 (509) | 71 (66) | 88 (85) | 68 (79) | 55 (74) | 42 (85) | 57 (94) |

# DECISIONS ABOUT FIELD OF PRACTICE 75

debt among doctors from low-income families was not significantly different from the frequency of such debt in all other doctors among the 1950 public school graduates, but in the 1954 public and the 1950 and 1954 private school graduates it was (CR range, 2.7–6.0).

Many medical students come from families of a high average income, but this must be balanced against the fact that medical education is costly. The fact that expenditures for medical education cause problems for many students is attested to by the many reported sources of support, the frequency of part-time employment, and, for a few, the debts accumulated at the conclusion of their education.

Any given level of economic difficulty, however, may be perceived and reacted to differently by different individuals. On the assumption that students and, where applicable, their spouses would react differently to the demands of a medical education, several questions were asked about the extent to which students felt that the cost and demands of a medical education had produced serious deprivation of food, clothing, housing, and leisure. The following few paragraphs refer only to the doctors who reported that these human needs had been curtailed by the expenses of their education.

The doctors offered judgments about their condition as students which seem very realistic. Very few felt that they had been deprived of food. Overall, about 15 percent were dissatisfied with their housing as medical students. About a quarter felt deprivation with respect to clothing, and a third with respect to leisure. Doctors' wives apparently felt deprivation more strongly than did the doctors themselves. As reported by the doctors who were married while in medical school, nearly half of the wives felt that their leisure was inadequate, and a quarter that housing was inadequate. The wives of surgeons were reportedly more dissatisfied with their lot than other wives. Since surgeons prolong their training for practice more than any other type of doctor, one must conclude that this dissatisfaction had little effect on surgeon's decisions about training. General practitioners, who obtain the least training before going into practice, did not seem to have any greater dissatisfaction than any other groups of doctors. The selection of field of practice thus does not seem to be greatly influenced by how the doctor or his wife felt about the deprivation imposed by a medical education.

Doctors were also questioned about their deprivation with respect to less essential but important aspects of life, such as recreational activities, keeping up with current affairs, nonmedical reading. The largest proportion of students—nearly three quarters—stated that their nonmedical reading had been limited by the demands of a medical education. The demands of a medical school seemed to fall equally on the classes of 1950 and 1954, whether private or public. The internists stated more frequently than did the other doctors that their education had interfered with their nonmedical reading. Surgeons most frequently complained about their inability to keep up with current events. Perhaps these characterizations may be added to the large catalogue of differences in the personalities of surgeons and internists, with the latter possibly more interested in reading books and the former in reading newspapers. In any event, in general the feeling of deprivation did not seem to be very strongly associated with any particular type of practice subsequently selected by the doctors. Nor did the feelings of the doctor's spouse with respect to the effects on family life and recreation seem to have exerted any influence on the doctor's choice of a field of practice.

## Marital Status

The fact that a doctor is married before he enters medical school or while he is in the midst of his education may be important in determining his plans for the future. A higher proportion of students was married before entering medical school in 1950 than in 1954, a fact probably relating to the war and the different ages of the students entering in these two years (see Table 26). In both 1950 and 1954 a higher proportion of the public school students was married before entering medical school than was the case in the private schools. (CR 3.6 and 2.1) The proportion of students who married while in medical school increased between 1950 and 1954, in both the public and private medical schools. Whereas half or more of the private medical school graduates were single when they finished their education, only slightly over a third of the public school graduates remained single (CR 3.0 in 1950, 4.4 in 1954).

The fact that more public than private school students marry before beginning their medical education may have several explanations. The public medical school graduates are older at the time of entering school and this fact itself is very probably associated with more frequent marriage. It is possible that these students have greater obligations and therefore select the less costly public medical schools. It will be noted below that the training and careers of doctors who graduate from private schools are different from those who graduate from public medical schools. The fact that the greater proportion of private school graduates remains single until the conclusion of medical education may be associated with these differences.

In Table 26 the time of marriage is also examined in relation to the three most common fields of practice. It will be seen that

TABLE 26. Percentage distribution of doctors by marital status, field of practice, type of school, and year of graduation

| Marital status | 1950 | | | | 1954 | | | |
|---|---|---|---|---|---|---|---|---|
| | All doctors | General practice | Medicine | Surgery | All doctors | General practice | Medicine | Surgery |
| | | | | Public | | | | |
| Before medical school | 38 | 56 | 21 | 26 | 21 | 34 | 12 | 11 |
| During medical school | 24 | 25 | 23 | 30 | 42 | 40 | 39 | 53 |
| Single during medical school | 38 | 19 | 56 | 44 | 37 | 26 | 49 | 36 |
| Total | (334) | (116) | (52) | (50) | (498) | (164) | (75) | (64) |
| | | | | Private | | | | |
| Before medical school | 26 | 46 | 31 | 16 | 13 | 33 | 11 | 15 |
| During medical school | 25 | 33 | 15 | 32 | 32 | 35 | 32 | 29 |
| Single during medical school | 49 | 21 | 54 | 52 | 55 | 32 | 57 | 56 |
| Total | (430) | (61) | (74) | (94) | (509) | (40) | (105) | (122) |

# DECISIONS ABOUT FIELD OF PRACTICE

a larger proportion of the general practitioners were married before entering medical school than was the case of internists or surgeons. The proportion of general practitioners who were married before entering medical school was significantly higher than all other doctors in all groups (CR 3.6 and 2.8 for public school graduates of 1950 and 1954, respectively, and 4.2 and 2.0 for private school graduates).

General practitioners are not notably different from all other doctors with respect to marriage while in medical school. Since they married at a higher rate before entry and at about the same rate as other doctors while in medical school, far fewer were single at the time of graduation than was the case of all doctors or for internists and surgeons. Examination of the marital status of other types of doctors does not indicate that it was notably different from that of all doctors. General practitioners seem to be unique in frequency of marriage before entering medical school. It is possible that this is a cause and effect relationship, that doctors go into general practice because they have been married for a longer time. The probability of having children and the attendant increased responsibilities almost certainly increase as marriage is prolonged. These differences were still present in 1961. Slightly over 3 percent of general practitioners were unmarried, a figure well below that of the whole group. For all doctors the 1961 figures were 5 percent and 8 percent still single among public school graduates of 1950 and 1954, and 12 percent and 8 percent still single among private school graduates.

Doctors who were single at the conclusion of their medical education were asked why they had not married before graduation. Over half of these single doctors simply stated they had not found the desired mate. Between a quarter and one third stated that inadequate income had forced postponement of marriage. A similar number stated that they had not seriously considered it, whereas somewhat more than 10 percent gave lack of time as a consideration. The various reasons given for the postponement of marriage do not show any considerable or marked association with any particular type of subsequent field of practice selected by the doctors.

*Friendships and Career Choices*

In an attempt to determine whether medical students influence one another in their choice of internship, residencies, and field of practice, several questions were asked. (18, 26) One dealt with friendships within the medical school class; that is, each doctor was asked to indicate who his best friends in the class were. The second question sought to determine whether a doctor's best friend might be in another medical school class, or outside the medical school. A third question sought to determine which students in each class enjoyed the greatest respect; for this purpose each doctor was asked to indicate which students he would have turned to for help in academic matters. The complexity of the material produced precludes any possibility of presenting a detailed analysis of these data here. A few observations of general significance will, however, be dealt with.

Doctors reported overwhelmingly that their closest friends and associates in medical school were fellow members of their own class. On the basis of reported friendships it was possible to define groups of friends within each class. Such groups were made up of students who claimed friends and were also claimed by others within the group. Within these groups it was further possible to subdivide the members into several categories—leaders

# DECISIONS ABOUT FIELD OF PRACTICE 81

and central and peripheral members. Outside these groups were other doctors who were not members of any group (although they had friends and were claimed by other doctors as friends), and isolates, who claimed very few friends and were seldom claimed as friends.

This labor yielded rather few results. In general, the position in the friendship circles showed no association with the ultimate practice selected by the doctors. One exception was psychiatry. A larger proportion of psychiatrists were group leaders or central members of the group than was the case with doctors in any other type of practice, and there was no isolates among those who later became psychiatrists. Conversely, doctors who ultimately chose careers in teaching and research seemed to have been isolates more frequently than was the case with any other type of specialist.

Answers to the question as to which students would be sought out for help on academic matters were used to construct a scale related to the esteem or respect which the students enjoyed from their peers. The group of students who ultimately selected teaching or research as their life work were much more highly esteemed by fellow students than other specialty groups. This was true in both the public and private medical school classes.

## Hospital Training and Field of Practice

The hospital which the doctor selects for internship may be determined by the field of practice he has chosen to enter, or, on the contrary, a doctor may make a decision about what field of practice he intends to enter as a result of his experience during internship. There is also the possibility that he may change his plans as a result of training. The associations between training and field of practice should be examined with full realization that cause-and-effect relationships are difficult to delineate.

In Table 27 the types of internship obtained by the doctors in the sample are shown. A very high proportion of the public school graduates began their training with a rotating internship, whereas only a bare majority of the private school graduates did. The critical ratio for the 1950 public-private school difference is 3.3 and for 1954, 3.9. In contrast with public school graduates, a third or more of the private school graduates began their training with a straight medical or surgical internship. Predictably, these public-private differences are also significant—the critical ratio for 1950 is 3.1 and for 1954, 3.5. The "other" internship category is a heterogenous group including straight internships in pediatrics and obstetrics-gynecology, mixed internships, as well as other experiences. In both 1950 and 1954 "other" internships were selected more frequently by private school gradu-

TABLE 27. Percentage distribution of doctors by type of internship, type of school, and year of graduation

| Type of internship | Public | | Private | |
| --- | --- | --- | --- | --- |
| | 1950 | 1954 | 1950 | 1954 |
| Rotating | 87 | 90 | 54 | 53 |
| Medical | 4 | 6 | 22 | 21 |
| Surgical | 3 | 1 | 11 | 15 |
| Other | 3 | 1 | 11 | 9 |
| No response | 4 | 2 | 2 | 1 |
| Total | (334) | (498) | (430) | (509) |

ates. The critical ratios for these public-private school differences are also significant; that for 1950 is 2.7 and for 1954, 2.8.

In Table 28 the doctors who obtained rotating internships have been distributed according to the field of practice reported in 1961. In the public medical schools nearly 90 percent of all doctors reported rotating internships. General practitioners were not very different in this respect from their classmates who selected other fields of practice. In the private medical schools 14 and 8 percent of the doctors who graduated in 1950 and 1954, respectively, entered general practice, and about 90 percent of them began their training with a rotating internship. They were clearly different from all other private school graduates in this

TABLE 28. Percentage of doctors with rotating internship by field of practice, type of school, and year of graduation

| | Public | | Private | |
|---|---|---|---|---|
| | 1950 | 1954 | 1950 | 1954 |
| Field of practice | Rotating | Rotating | Rotating | Rotating |
| General practice | 96 (114) | 99 (160) | 90 (59) | 90 (40) |
| Medicine | 80 (49) | 80 (75) | 44 (73) | 55 (104) |
| Surgery | 86 (50) | 95 (64) | 51 (92) | 47 (120) |
| Pediatrics | 80 (15) | 87 (23) | 53 (34) | 56 (41) |
| Obstetrics-gynecology | 90 (10) | 94 (32) | 62 (26) | 80 (25) |
| Psychiatry | 92 (24) | 81 (32) | 49 (33) | 56 (34) |
| Teaching and research | 89 (18) | 78 (36) | 32 (56) | 25 (84) |
| Other | 95 (41) | 92 (65) | 68 (38) | 71 (49) |
| Not in practice | 100 (1) | 67 (3) | 80 (10) | 60 (5) |
| All doctors | 90 (322) | 91 (490) | 56 (421) | 54 (502) |

respect (CR for this difference was 4.4 for 1950 classes and 3.5 for 1954 classes). The distribution of men in other fields of practice who had rotating internships is quite similar to the distribution of all graduates, although men who enter obstetrics-gynecology are more like general practitioners in their tendency to begin training with a rotating internship, and men who enter teaching and research are least likely to do so. The difference between the doctors reporting obstetrics-gynecology practices in 1961 and all other specialists with respect to the rotating internship was significant only for 1954 private school graduates (CR 2.0). The teachers and researchers who graduated in 1954 were significantly different from doctors in all other fields of practice (CR 2.3 for public and 2.4 for private school graduates) because of the infrequency with which they reported a rotating internship. The teachers and researchers were not significantly different from other 1950 graduates, whether of a public or a private school. Overall, nearly half of the private school graduates who went into specialty practice began their training with a rotating internship, but an even higher proportion of the public school specialists did so, and this difference was significant both in 1950 (CR 3.1) and 1954 (CR 3.2).

A substantially larger proportion of the private school graduates obtained their internship in a major teaching hospital than was the case with the public school graduates (see Table 29). The critical ratio for this difference was 2.5 for the 1950 classes to 2.3 for the 1954 classes. The hospital of internship is also shown in Table 29 in relation to certain fields of practice. It will be noted that among both the private and public school graduates of 1950 and 1954 a smaller proportion of the general practitioners reported major teaching hospital internships than was the case of doctors in the other fields shown; this difference was

TABLE 29. Percentage distribution of doctors by hospital of internship, all doctors and by field of practice, by type of school and year of graduation

| Hospital of internship | 1950 | | | | | 1954 | | | | |
|---|---|---|---|---|---|---|---|---|---|---|
| | All doctors | General practice | Medicine | Surgery | Teaching and research | All doctors | General practice | Medicine | Surgery | Teaching and research |
| Public | | | | | | | | | | |
| Major teaching | 40 | 28 | 56 | 38 | 63 | 42 | 31 | 60 | 36 | 50 |
| Other | 60 | 72 | 44 | 62 | 32 | 58 | 68 | 40 | 63 | 45 |
| No response | 1 | 1 | 0 | 0 | 5 | 1 | 0 | 0 | 2 | 5 |
| | (334) | (116) | (52) | (50) | (19) | (498) | (164) | (75) | (64) | (38) |
| Private | | | | | | | | | | |
| Major teaching | 65 | 31 | 76 | 67 | 85 | 70 | 38 | 74 | 68 | 92 |
| Other | 35 | 69 | 24 | 33 | 12 | 30 | 63 | 26 | 32 | 7 |
| No response | 1 | 0 | 0 | 0 | 3 | 0 | 0 | 0 | 0 | 1 |
| | (430) | (61) | (74) | (94) | (59) | (509) | (40) | (105) | (122) | (86) |

significant for both public (CR 2.4) and private (CR 3.1) school graduates of 1950, but not for those of 1954. In three of the four groups the doctors whose careers were in the field of teaching and research had obtained major teaching hospital internships in a substantially higher proportion than that of any of the other groups shown. The differences between this small group and all others was significant only for the private school graduates (CR 2.5 for 1950 and 2.2 for 1954 classes). The critical ratio for the corresponding public school comparison was borderline, 1.9 for the 1950 classes, and not significant for the 1954 classes. The other specialties, such as pediatrics, psychiatry, and obstetrics-gynecology, were not notably different from surgeons and internists. The proportion of general practitioners with a major teaching hospital internship is very similar in both years and also among private and public medical school graduates. This is in rather sharp contrast to the experience of the specialist group. The specialists who graduated from private medical schools obtained major teaching hospital internships substantially more frequently than was the case of those graduating from public schools (CR 2.5 for 1950 graduates and 1.8 for 1954 classes).

Residency training was quite similar to internship in its relationship to field of practice (See Table 30). The proportion of physicians for whom there was "No Response" is virtually identical with the proportion who had no residency. The proportion of doctors who obtained residencies increased from 70 to 75 percent between 1950 and 1954 among the public (CR 2.5) and from 90 to 96 percent among private medical school graduates (CR 4.1).

The proportion of doctors who proceeded to residency varied substantially with the field of practice pursued. Only about a quarter of the public school graduates who went into general

TABLE 30. Percentage distribution of doctors by hospital of residency, all doctors and by field of practice, by type of school, and year of graduation

| Hospital of residency | 1950 | | | | | 1954 | | | | |
|---|---|---|---|---|---|---|---|---|---|---|
| | All doctors | General practice | Medicine | Surgery | Teaching and research | All doctors | General practice | Medicine | Surgery | Teaching and research |
| *Public* | | | | | | | | | | |
| Major teaching | 24 | 4 | 39 | 20 | 42 | 32 | 7 | 33 | 33 | 71 |
| Other | 46 | 17 | 58 | 80 | 42 | 43 | 27 | 60 | 66 | 21 |
| No response | 30 | 79 | 4 | 0 | 16 | 25 | 67 | 3 | 2 | 8 |
| | (334) | (116) | (52) | (50) | (19) | (498) | (164) | (75) | (64) | (38) |
| *Private* | | | | | | | | | | |
| Major teaching | 40 | 12 | 47 | 45 | 56 | 46 | 20 | 37 | 43 | 70 |
| Other | 52 | 56 | 50 | 54 | 34 | 50 | 48 | 63 | 57 | 27 |
| No response | 9 | 33 | 3 | 1 | 10 | 4 | 33 | 0 | 0 | 3 |
| | (498) | (61) | (74) | (94) | (59) | (509) | (40) | (105) | (122) | (86) |

practice obtained any residency whereas two thirds of the general practitioners who graduated from private schools continued their training beyond the internship; this difference was significant (CR 8.3 and 5.0 in 1950 and 1954).

When public school graduates alone are considered, the general practitioners have a strikingly higher frequency of obtaining no residency training as compared to all other public school graduates in both 1950 (CR 20.5) and 1954 (CR 24.2). In private schools also general practitioners are much more likely than all other doctors to obtain no residency (CR 6.5 and 5.7 in 1950 and 1954).

When all doctors (without regard to field of practice) are considered with respect to residency training, another striking difference between public and private schools appears, as shown in Table 30. A higher proportion of the private school group reported major teaching hospital residency, and this difference from public school graduates was significant (CR 2.0) in both 1950 and 1954.

Among public school graduates, general practitioners were significantly less likely to report major teaching hospital residencies as compared to all other doctors (CR 4.0 and 8.6 in 1950 and 1954), and the same difference is found among private school graduates (CR 4.9 and 2.4 in 1950 and 1954). Finally, as shown in Table 31, the likelihood of reporting residency training of

TABLE 31. Percent of doctors reporting 24 months or more residency training

|  | 1950 | 1954 |
| --- | --- | --- |
| Public | 61 (205) | 65 (322) |
| Private | 90 (350) | 87 (445) |

two years or more duration was significantly higher in private than in public schools (CR 4.6 in 1950, 4.8 in 1954).

Almost all of these differences in residency training between public and private schools are, in fact, due to the general practitioners. When general practitioners are eliminated from consideration, no significant differences between public and private schools is found with regard to physicians reporting no residency training and with regard to physicians reporting residency in a major teaching hospital. In other words, the residency training of specialists does not seem to vary significantly between public and private schools.

The doctors who selected to go into fields other than general practice almost universally obtained residency training (Table 32). The length of the residency training for general practitioners was short—averaging eighteen months—compared with an average of thirty-six months for all other doctors except pediatricians, whose average was slightly over two years. The pediatricians as a group obtained a residency training in a major teaching hospital in about the same proportion as did other specialist groups even though their average period of residency was shorter. Doctors engaged in teaching and research, who had major teaching hospital residency more frequently than did all other doctors, reported no residency somewhat more frequently than other specialists. Naturally, they reported more nonclinical training than other specialists.

*Academic Achievement and Field of Practice*

The Medical College Admission Test (MCAT), which presumably measures both knowledge and ability, has been widely used as part of the selection process for medical schools. Its utility as a predictor of performance in medical school has been

TABLE 32. Percent of doctors with residency and average duration of residency by field of practice and type of school (1950 and 1954 combined)

| Field of practice | Public | | Private | |
|---|---|---|---|---|
| | Percent with residency | Average duration (months) | Percent with residency | Average duration (months) |
| General practice | 28 (280) | 18 | 66 (101) | 18 |
| Medicine | 97 (127) | 37 | 99 (179) | 36 |
| Surgery | 100 (114) | 44 | 99 (216) | 47 |
| Teaching and research | 89 (57) | 37 | 94 (145) | 33 |
| Psychiatry | 95 (57) | 37 | 100 (68) | 41 |
| Pediatrics | 100 (38) | 27 | 96 (76) | 27 |
| Obstetrics-gynecology | 100 (44) | 39 | 100 (51) | 40 |
| Eye, ear, nose, throat | 98 (44) | 33 | 100 (26) | 37 |
| Pathology | 100 (20) | 47 | 100 (22) | 40 |
| Radiology | 100 (31) | 38 | 100 (26) | 40 |

debatable. In some medical schools it apparently does not show any association with academic performance, whereas in others it shows weak correlations. However, it appears that this test has interesting attributes in relation to career decisions, as is shown in Table 33. The 1950 graduates did not take this test so the experience of only 1954 graduates is shown, and, of course, these figures do not include students who were admitted to medical school in 1954 but failed or withdrew.

Although a difference between public and private schools in the distribution of MCAT scores among all doctors might be suspected on examination of Table 32, no significant difference between public and private schools was, in fact, found on statistical analysis. Indeed, detailed examination of the data revealed that almost all of the apparent overrepresentation of high MCAT scores among private schools (as compared to public schools) was traceable to the scores of students at just three schools—all of which have a history of producing teachers and researchers and all of which happen to be private.

In both the public and the private schools the proportion of general practitioners with low MCAT scores was large and the proportion of general practitioners was correspondingly

TABLE 33. Percent of doctors by field of practice, by composite MCAT score and type of school (1954 graduates)

| | MCAT | | | | | |
| | Public | | | Private | | |
| Field of practice | -500 | 501-600 | 601- | -500 | 501-600 | 601- |
|---|---|---|---|---|---|---|
| All doctors | 28 | 53 | 19 | 17 | 42 | 41 |
| General practice | 43 | 28 | 23 | 12 | 8 | 7 |
| Medicine | 12 | 15 | 23 | 19 | 21 | 20 |
| Surgery | 15 | 15 | 6 | 27 | 30 | 16 |
| Teaching and research | 4 | 7 | 13 | 7 | 9 | 28 |
| Psychiatry | 4 | 8 | 8 | 0 | 7 | 10 |
| Pediatrics | 5 | 5 | 5 | 12 | 6 | 8 |
| Other | 18 | 22 | 23 | 22 | 19 | 10 |
| | (127) | (238) | (87) | (81) | (203) | (201) |

smaller in the high score group; when this relationship was tested by a calculation of the regression, it was found to be significant (CR 2.2) for the public school group.

In the public schools there was twice as large a proportion of internists with high MCAT scores as there was in the lowest group (CR of the regression, 2.6), but this distribution was not apparent among private school students who became internists. If the internists whose principal activity was teaching or research are combined with those in private practice the picture with respect to the public school group is not altered. This redistribution has an effect on the private school graduate internists. The percentages with low, middle, and high scores become 23, 26, and 35 percent, respectively. This is the only field of practice affected by this redistribution. As mentioned in the methods section, a similar redistribution of the teaching and research group has been performed to test its effect on all major tables. With the exception of the changes shown above and some effect on class rank distributions, it has produced no alterations of importance. Doctors engaged in teaching and research were definitely selected from among the students with high scores. In private schools this was significant (CR of the regression, 7.2), but it did not reach significance in the public schools (CR of the regression, 1.7), probably because of the effect of small numbers and high variance.

It is well recognized that class rank in medical school is important in determining what kind of an internship the graduate obtains. The type of internship is, in turn, likely to be related to subsequent training and to what the doctor does when his training is finished. When the relationship between class rank in medical school and subsequent selection of a field of practice is examined, three effects are found (Table 34). Doctors who en-

TABLE 34. Percentage distribution of doctors by field of practice, class rank, type of school, and year of graduation

| Field of practice | Class rank | | | | | |
|---|---|---|---|---|---|---|
| | Public | | | Private | | |
| | Lower | Middle | Upper | Lower | Middle | Upper |
| | | | 1950 | | | |
| General practice | 41 | 41 | 23 | 21 | 15 | 7 |
| Medicine | 11 | 10 | 26 | 14 | 13 | 25 |
| Teaching and research | 2 | 3 | 12 | 6 | 17 | 18 |
| Surgery | 14 | 17 | 15 | 27 | 24 | 17 |
| Psychiatry | 12 | 3 | 7 | 10 | 7 | 6 |
| Pediatrics | 2 | 7 | 5 | 4 | 12 | 8 |
| Obstetrics-gynecology | 7 | 2 | 2 | 7 | 5 | 6 |
| Other | 13 | 16 | 11 | 10 | 6 | 12 |
| | (103) | (119) | (110) | (135) | (139) | (146) |
| | | | 1954 | | | |
| General practice | 46 | 38 | 16 | 13 | 8 | 2 |
| Medicine | 5 | 13 | 27 | 17 | 19 | 26 |
| Teaching and research | 6 | 7 | 10 | 11 | 14 | 25 |
| Surgery | 18 | 9 | 14 | 24 | 26 | 22 |
| Psychiatry | 6 | 7 | 6 | 11 | 5 | 5 |
| Pediatrics | 5 | 5 | 3 | 7 | 10 | 8 |
| Obstetrics-gynecology | 5 | 7 | 7 | 6 | 5 | 3 |
| Other | 9 | 13 | 18 | 10 | 11 | 8 |
| | (147) | (193) | (155) | (164) | (166) | (174) |

ter certain fields of practice are recruited from all segments of their class, high, middle, or low rank, without distinction. Doctors who select other fields of practice are recruited mainly from the bottom portion of the class. A third group is recruited from the top part of the class.

The surgeons are an example of the first distribution; they are drawn from all parts of the class without any evidence of systematic selection. The general practitioners were clearly drawn in disproportionate numbers from the lowest third of the class. In the public schools the proportion of general practitioners drawn from the top part of the class was less than half the proportion drawn from the bottom. Among the private school graduates three times as many general practitioners ranked in the lowest third as in the upper third of the class. When these relationships are examined statistically, by a calculation of the significance of the regressions, the inverse relationship between class rank and selection of general practice is found to be significant in public schools (CR 3.2 and 4.9) as well as in private schools (CR 2.5 and 4.2) in both 1950 and 1954.

Internists were drawn in excess from among the more able medical students as measured by class rank. In the case of the public school graduates three times as many internists ranked in the top third of their class as in the bottom; although the effect is not so marked among the private school graduates, it is still quite definite. This positive relationship between class rank and selection of internal medicine was significant in every case except in public schools in 1950.

Doctors who reported that they were engaged in teaching and research show a relationship to class rank similar to that of internists. The proportion of teachers and researchers that ranked in the top third of the class was between two to three times as great as the proportion ranking in the bottom third. This positive relationship between class rank and selection of teaching and research was significant in both public (CR 3.6) and private (CR 2.1) schools in 1950, but in neither case in 1954.

*Decisions about Training*

A doctor's decision to be a general practitioner or a specialist or to go into research has implications with respect to how he will train. Whatever field of practice the doctor selects, he presumably must decide how much and what kind of training he wants. Some of these decisions will be under his control and others will not. He may decide that he wants a rotating internship, and it is very probable that he will obtain one. He may decide to intern in a major teaching hospital, but this decision is one which he may not be able to realize.

The doctors who participated in this study were asked a series of questions relating to their decisions. The first question sought to determine if the student was encouraged to continue his training beyond the internship by his family and spouse (who might be affected by such a decision) or by his academic or clinical teachers (who might have a more disinterested point of view). In an attempt to determine whether such advice was important or unimportant, the doctors were asked if they could identify any person whose advice proved to be decisive in helping them to make choices about hospital training. A third question dealt with the time at which the decision about the doctor's hospital training was made. This is an important question if the thesis that longer training is associated with greater clinical competence is correct. For example, if it were considered desirable to influence more future students toward longer training, it would be important to know whether decisions about training usually are made in medical school or at a later time. Lastly, the doctors were asked how much training had been decided upon.

About one in ten doctors made his decision about the amount of training he intended to obtain before entering medical school (Table 35). About a quarter of the public school graduates made their decisions when they were in medical school. About a third of the private school graduates made the decision while they were taking their internship. Quite a few doctors did not finally decide this matter until they reached the residency training period.

The timing of the doctor's decision with respect to his training varied with his field of practice. The largest proportion of general practitioners—about half—made their decision during the internship. This difference between general practitioners and all other doctors was significant in every case except for private schools in 1954 (a group in which the number of general practitioners was small). This finding suggests that something about the internship was involved; it may be that the doctor discovered that his finances were insufficient, or that he found it difficult to obtain residency appointments. The internists and surgeons did not show any characteristic pattern with respect to timing of the decision about training. There was a tendency for this decision to be made by both groups while still in medical school, although many did not make the decision until they were interns or even in their residency training. Doctors who selected careers in teaching and research tended to make their decision very early: In the various groups 37 to 55 percent reported that they had made the decision during or before medical school.

A summary of the information supplied by all doctors and by general practitioners on the amount of training they decided to

TABLE 35. Percentage distribution of all doctors by time of final training decision and by field of practice, type of school, and year of graduation

| Time of decision | 1950 | | | | | | 1954 | | | | | |
|---|---|---|---|---|---|---|---|---|---|---|---|---|
| | All doctors | General practice | Medicine | Surgery | Teaching and research | | All doctors | General practice | Medicine | Surgery | Teaching and research | |
| | | | | | | Public | | | | | | |
| Before medical school | 8 | 15 | 0 | 4 | 5 | | 8 | 9 | 4 | 6 | 13 | |
| During medical school | 27 | 26 | 33 | 32 | 32 | | 27 | 30 | 19 | 27 | 32 | |
| While intern | 40 | 50 | 38 | 26 | 26 | | 42 | 49 | 49 | 36 | 29 | |
| While resident | 16 | 5 | 17 | 22 | 16 | | 16 | 9 | 24 | 23 | 24 | |
| Other | 9 | 3 | 10 | 16 | 21 | | 6 | 2 | 4 | 8 | 3 | |
| No response | 1 | 1 | 2 | 0 | 0 | | 0 | 1 | 0 | 0 | 0 | |
| | (334) | (116) | (52) | (50) | (19) | | (498) | (164) | (75) | (64) | (38) | |
| | | | | | | Private | | | | | | |
| Before medical school | 9 | 2 | 7 | 11 | 8 | | 10 | 5 | 3 | 17 | 13 | |
| During medical school | 32 | 13 | 49 | 35 | 37 | | 35 | 28 | 31 | 37 | 42 | |
| While intern | 33 | 54 | 23 | 33 | 24 | | 26 | 35 | 28 | 23 | 14 | |
| While resident | 23 | 30 | 19 | 19 | 31 | | 26 | 25 | 33 | 20 | 31 | |
| Other | 2 | 0 | 3 | 1 | 0 | | 3 | 8 | 4 | 2 | 0 | |
| No response | 1 | 2 | 0 | 1 | 0 | | 0 | 0 | 1 | 1 | 0 | |
| | (430) | (61) | (74) | (94) | (59) | | (509) | (40) | (105) | (122) | (86) | |

undertake is shown in Table 36. The differences between public and private school graduates were striking. For example, considering all doctors, a much larger proportion decided on internship only in the public than in the private schools (CR 9.0 and 5.1) in both 1950 and 1954. Conversely, a significantly larger proportion of private school than public school graduates decided on certification in both years (CR 4.1 and 4.6).

TABLE 36. Percentage distribution of all doctors and general practitioners by amount of training decided upon, type of school, and year of graduation

| | All doctors | | | | General practitioners | | | |
|---|---|---|---|---|---|---|---|---|
| | Public | | Private | | Public | | Private | |
| Amount of training | 1950 | 1954 | 1950 | 1954 | 1950 | 1954 | 1950 | 1954 |
| Internship only | 29 | 23 | 7 | 4 | 76 | 64 | 28 | 32 |
| Partial residency | 11 | 11 | 12 | 8 | 22 | 32 | 57 | 58 |
| Sufficient for board certification | 60 | 65 | 80 | 88 | 2 | 4 | 15 | 10 |
| | (333) | (498) | (429) | (508) | (116) | (164) | (61) | (40) |

There is, of course, many a slip 'twixt the cup and the lip, so that the proportion of doctors actually certified is less than those who intended to obtain qualification. At the time this study was done, in 1961, it was clear that the 1950 graduates who were to be certified had completed the process, whereas the 1954 graduates were still obtaining certification. Among the 1950 graduates 60 percent of the public school graduates indicated in 1961 that they intended to become certified. By 1960, 26 to 50 percent of the graduates of the various schools had actually achieved it.

Whereas 80 percent of the 1950 private school graduates indicated in 1961 that they were going to obtain sufficient residency for certification, 40 to 68 percent of the graduates of the different schools were certified by 1961.

When general practitioners alone are considered, it is clear that—in contrast with all other physicians—a much higher proportion originally intended to obtain internship only (CR of the difference ranged from 3.3 to 23.7 in public and private schools in 1950 and 1954). Similarly, far fewer general practitioners than other doctors planned to obtain partial residency (CR ranged from 4.8 to 10) and certification (CR range, 13.8 to 45).

In almost every instance—regarding internship only, partial residency, or certification—there was a significant public school–private school difference among general practitioners, with private school graduates planning to obtain more training than their public school counterparts. The difference in proportion of public and private school graduates in general practice who decided to limit training to internship only was significant in both 1950 (CR 9.8) and 1954 (CR 3.2). Decisions involving a partial residency were also significantly different between the public and private school graduates who entered general practice (CR 5.4 for 1950 and 2.8 for 1954 classes). The number of general practitioners who had decided to obtain certification was small; nevertheless the public–private difference was significant in 1950 (CR 2.3). In contrast, when general practitioners are ignored and all other doctors are examined with regard to plans for internship only, partial residency, or certification, no consistent difference between public and private schools is found.

Table 37 shows the proportion of doctors who reported that they were encouraged to continue their training beyond the internship and by whom. The private school graduates received

TABLE 37. Percent of doctors reporting encouragement in planning training by people influencing training beyond internship, all doctors, by field of practice, year of graduation, and type of school

| | All doctors | | General practitioners | | Medicine | | Surgery | | Teaching and research | |
|---|---|---|---|---|---|---|---|---|---|---|
| | 1950 | 1954 | 1950 | 1954 | 1950 | 1954 | 1950 | 1954 | 1950 | 1954 |
| | | | | | Public | | | | | |
| Parents | 24 | 26 | 8 | 15 | 35 | 32 | 42 | 41 | 26 | 45 |
| Spouse | 34 | 36 | 12 | 18 | 44 | 44 | 50 | 48 | 42 | 34 |
| Medical school teachers | 38 | 47 | 34 | 38 | 50 | 63 | 34 | 36 | 47 | 61 |
| Dean or adviser | 17 | 18 | 13 | 15 | 27 | 27 | 16 | 13 | 32 | 29 |
| Clinical chiefs | 48 | 55 | 41 | 45 | 58 | 71 | 54 | 61 | 53 | 50 |
| Attending physician | 40 | 49 | 33 | 38 | 44 | 65 | 46 | 58 | 21 | 32 |
| Residents | 36 | 46 | 26 | 36 | 50 | 61 | 46 | 47 | 42 | 42 |
| Personal physician | 13 | 13 | 9 | 15 | 13 | 15 | 12 | 5 | 16 | 13 |
| Other | 7 | 6 | – | – | – | – | – | – | – | – |
| | (334) | (498) | (116) | (164) | (52) | (75) | (50) | (64) | (19) | (38) |

TABLE 37 (Continued)

|  | All doctors | | General practitioners | | Private Medicine | | Surgery | | Teaching and research | |
|---|---|---|---|---|---|---|---|---|---|---|
|  | 1950 | 1954 | 1950 | 1954 | 1950 | 1954 | 1950 | 1954 | 1950 | 1954 |
| Parents | 38 | 45 | 15 | 30 | 39 | 48 | 45 | 57 | 41 | 34 |
| Spouse | 47 | 47 | 36 | 33 | 50 | 45 | 52 | 54 | 36 | 48 |
| Medical school teachers | 54 | 62 | 43 | 70 | 61 | 65 | 56 | 58 | 66 | 67 |
| Dean or adviser | 29 | 40 | 30 | 53 | 24 | 47 | 35 | 43 | 34 | 40 |
| Clinical chiefs | 65 | 68 | 61 | 60 | 70 | 71 | 73 | 75 | 61 | 71 |
| Attending physician | 65 | 62 | 52 | 55 | 74 | 70 | 77 | 67 | 58 | 57 |
| Residents | 61 | 63 | 48 | 63 | 64 | 70 | 67 | 66 | 59 | 65 |
| Personal physician | 18 | 19 | 13 | 18 | 11 | 15 | 20 | 28 | 5 | 13 |
| Other | 10 | 8 | — | — | — | — | — | — | — | — |
|  | (430) | (509) | (61) | (40) | (74) | (105) | (84) | (122) | (59)1 | (86) |

more encouragement from all sources than did the public school graduates. This was true whether the source of the advice was parents, spouse, teachers, or personal physicians, and the difference was significant in almost every case. More doctors reported that they were encouraged by their clinical chiefs than by anyone else. A personal physician seems to have been a rare source of encouragement, and parents and spouse only a minor source. Medical school deans or student advisers, whose duties presumably include student guidance, seem to have seldom provided encouragement. In addition to receiving advice from a clinical chief, the doctors seem to be advised by other clinical teachers, junior and senior, with considerable frequency. This is probably to be expected; it is when the doctor has contact with these people that he will be thinking about his decision. It is also at this time that he will be displaying the characteristics that may invite advice and encouragement, or, on the contrary, stony silence.

When the encouragement given to physicians to continue their training beyond the internship is examined by field of practice, rather marked differences are found. The general practitioners, as a group, received less encouragement to continue their training than did all doctors, or doctors who went into specialty practice. Whereas a quarter to nearly a half of all doctors in the various groups reported that their parents had encouraged them, the corresponding figures for general practitioners varied from 8 percent to a maximum of 30 percent. This difference was significant in public schools in both years and in private schools in 1950. General practitioners' spouses encouraged them less frequently than did the spouses of all other doctors, and this was significant in both public and private schools in both years (CR range 3.3 to 8). Medical school teachers, clinical chiefs, and other clinical teachers also seemed to give general practitioners relatively little backing, but these differences reached significance only irregularly.

The doctors who were practicing internal medicine, in general, received somewhat more encouragement from all sources than did all other doctors, but, again, differences between internists and others in this respect were only occasionally significant. This includes both advice received from family and from medical school and clinical teachers. Surgeons consistently reported greater encouragement from their parents and spouses. The amount of enouragement which they received from their preclinical and clinical teachers seems to have been variable. Doctors who pursued careers in teaching and research seemed to have received more encouragement from their medical school teachers and their deans and advisers than did other students. They were not consistently different from all physicians in respect to receiving advice from clinical chiefs.

When the data from the individual schools is examined, quite consistent differences emerge. A majority of the students among all of the private school graduates reported that they were urged to continue their training by their clinical chiefs, attending physicians, and residents. Among the public school graduates less encouragement was reported. The clinical chiefs were the major source of encouragement to continue training; in some of the schools less than half of the students reported that they had received encouragement from this source. This group of students received very little encouragement, on the whole, from attending physicians and residents in making their future plans.

# V / Hospital Training Decisions

WHILE IT IS CLEAR that the family, social, and economic backgrounds of doctors—discussed in the previous chapter—are important influences in a physician's subsequent career choices, the interrelated processes of selecting a field of practice and preparing for it are not determined only or even mainly by the doctor's early background. Hospital training is of major importance, and should be examined in detail to show how it is related to the doctor's background and to his selected field of practice.

*Influences Reported by Doctors on Decisions about a
Field of Practice and Their Relation to Training*

We have seen that selections of internship were quite different among public and private school graduates in the samples. Between 80 and 90 percent of the former in both 1950 and 1954 reported rotating internships, whereas a bare majority—54 and 53 percent—of the private school graduates reported rotating internships. About one third of private school graduates reported straight medical or surgical internships; in addition, they reported substantially more "other" preliminary training programs, including other straight internships and various types of postgraduate work. This difference between public and private school graduates was significant in both 1950 and 1954 (CR range from 3.1 to 3.9).

It will be recalled that doctors were asked to what extent their intellectual interests, interests in certain types of patients, finances, social circumstances, spouses' demands, or other pressures affected their choice of a field of practice. Doctors who stated that their practice decisions were influenced substantially by one or another of these factors will be examined here to see if, and how much, such influences were associated with various types of internships and residencies, and whether the length of training was affected.

As described in Chapter IV, most doctors reported that their intellectual interests were important in selecting a career. This was especially marked in the case of doctors who chose internal medicine or teaching and research. General practitioners, pediatricians, and obstetrician-gynecologists were influenced more than other doctors by interest in patients. General practitioners reported that social pressures or the influence of a spouse were important more frequently than did other doctors. Did these influences on choice of a field of practice have any relationship to the type of internship chosen? This question is examined in Table 38. Doctors who obtained straight internships reported that their intellectual interests were an important influence in selecting their field of practice more frequently than did those who reported rotating training. This difference was significant (CR range from 2.1 to 3.9) for all groups except the private school graduates of 1954 for whom the critical ratio was borderline (1.9).

Doctors who had had a rotating internship reported that finances were important to their decisions about practice more frequently than did those who had had a straight internship. Since the rotating internship often terminates formal training, and straight service internships usually are followed by more training, the association appears to be a very straightforward one. The difference was significant only for the 1950 private school classes (CR 3.2) and the 1954 public school graduates (CR

TABLE 38. Percent of doctors strongly influenced in choice of field of practice, by influential factor, type of internship, type of school, and year of graduation

| Influential factors | Public | | | | | | 1950 | | 1954 | |
|---|---|---|---|---|---|---|---|---|---|---|
| | 1950 | | 1954 | | | | Rotating | Straight Medical/ Surgical | Rotating | Straight Medical/ Surgical |
| | Rotating | Straight Medical/ Surgical | Rotating | Straight Medical/ Surgical | | | | | | |
| Intellectual | 75 (271) | 86 (21) | 75 (436) | 86 (37) | | | 80 (225) | 89 (140) | 85 (265) | 92 (184) |
| Financial | 33 (262) | 24 (21) | 25 (430) | 6 (35) | | | 26 (207) | 13 (125) | 15 (252) | 9 (175) |
| Patient interest | 40 (259) | 19 (21) | 38 (426) | 23 (35) | | | 37 (209) | 27 (123) | 30 (251) | 22 (175) |

4.5). There was little significant difference beween public and private schools in relation to this finding.

The distribution of doctors influenced by identification with certain types of patients was rather similar to that of doctors reporting they were influenced by finances, with more interest in patients reported by those who chose rotating internships. The differences in this respect among public school graduates were definite (CR 2.8 for the 1950 classes and 4.1 for the 1954 classes), but were not significant for the private school groups.

Selections of a hospital for internship also appeared to be associated with the factors that were influences upon a choice of a practice field (Table 39). Doctors who interned in major teaching hospitals consistently reported that they were influenced by their intellectual interest more frequently than those who interned in other hospitals. These differences were significant only for the private school graduates (CR 2.2 for the 1950 classes and 2.0 for 1954). A higher percentage of doctors who interned in other hospitals reported that financial considerations were important. This difference was definite among the public school classes of 1950 (CR 2.5) and the private school graduates of 1954 (CR 3.6), borderline (CR 1.99) for the 1950 private school graduates, and not significant for 1954 public school classes. No consistent association was evident when influences such as social pressure or a discontented spouse—which were important to fewer doctors—were examined.

It is important to recognize, of course, that we are dealing with more than the choice of hospital by our respondents when we examine doctors who interned in major teaching hospitals or other hospitals; there is also choice of intern by the hospitals involved, and our respondents did not have unilateral control over their internship placements. We do not have data on all

TABLE 39. Percent of doctors strongly influenced in choice of field of practice by influential factor and by hospital of internship

| Influential factor | Public | | | | Private | | | |
|---|---|---|---|---|---|---|---|---|
| | 1950 | | 1954 | | 1950 | | 1954 | |
| | Major teaching | All others | Major teaching | All others | Major teaching | All others | Major teaching | All others |
| Intellectual | 78 | 67 | 78 | 71 | 84 | 74 | 90 | 81 |
| Finance | 21 | 34 | 20 | 25 | 14 | 25 | 8 | 18 |
| Social | 17 | 23 | 17 | 13 | 8 | 17 | 9 | 12 |
| | (132) | (199) | (210) | (285) | (278) | (149) | (354) | (154) |

the internship applications made by our respondents; in short, we are dealing not so much with internship preference as with internship outcome. The assumption is made that outcome—where a doctor interns—is related to his preferences.

The doctors who went on to residency were a selected group, so it would be anticipated that any associations between residency choice and the reported influences affecting career choices would be weaker. This proved to be the case. Table 40 illustrates

TABLE 40. Percent of doctors strongly influenced in choice of field of practice, by influential factor and months of residency, by type of school, and by year of graduation

| Influential factor | Months of residency | | | | | | | |
|---|---|---|---|---|---|---|---|---|
| | Public | | | | Private | | | |
| | None | 1-23 | 24-47 | 48- | None | 1-23 | 24-47 | 48- |
| | | | | 1950 | | | | |
| Intellectual | 52 | 66 | 82 | 81 | 68 | 70 | 81 | 88 |
| Finances | 62 | 34 | 11 | 14 | 51 | 33 | 14 | 10 |
| Social | 37 | 21 | 12 | 14 | 32 | 33 | 8 | 5 |
| Spouse | 41 | 10 | 8 | 8 | 27 | 21 | 7 | 7 |
| | (100) | (29) | (142) | (63) | (37) | (43) | (239) | (111) |
| | | | | 1954 | | | | |
| Intellectual | 50 | 70 | 82 | 89 | 76 | 74 | 87 | 92 |
| Finances | 53 | 26 | 10 | 12 | 57 | 19 | 8 | 9 |
| Social | 26 | 17 | 10 | 8 | 33 | 26 | 5 | 10 |
| Spouse | 22 | 9 | 7 | 5 | 29 | 19 | 6 | 8 |
| | (123) | (53) | (239) | (83) | (21) | (43) | (278) | (167) |

the reports of doctors who obtained no residency, or varying amounts of residency, as to the factors influencing their choice of a field of practice. This table includes only the 1950 public school graduates, but the responses of all graduates, whether of public or private schools in 1950 or 1954, were very similar.

Doctors who obtained moderately long or long periods of residency training gave greater weight to their intellectual interests in selecting a field of practice than did those with shorter training. Among those who obtained no residency fewer claimed this interest than was the case among doctors with residency training. The difference in intellectual interest between the doctors reporting residency and no residency was highly significant for the public school graduates of both 1950 (CR 4.5) and 1954 (CR 6.1). The fact that the private school differences were not significant is undoubtedly related to the small numbers who did not obtain any residency, 37 in 1950 and 31 in 1954.

When doctors with no residency are compared with doctors who obtained residency training as to their reports of influence by financial factors, striking differences appear within both the public school and the private school groups. Among public school graduates, physicians with no residency reported financial influences much more frequently than doctors who reported some residency (CR 6.0 and 5.3 in 1950 and 1954), and the same is true within the private schools (CR 3.2 and 4.2 in 1950 and 1954). When all physicians who obtained residency training were considered, there was no difference between public and private school graduates in reporting financial influences; and no public-private school difference in reporting financial influences was found among all physicians with no residency. Thus, it is clear that the extremely significant association between financial factors and residency training overrides the usual pattern of public-private school differences, and that a major factor in all cases is the financial pressure—or lack of it—on graduates weighing residency choices.

This same pattern obtains for the influence of social pressures and spouse on residency. With marked significance (CR range 2.2 to 10.4) physicians with no residency reported these influences more frequently, and this occurred both in public and private schools.

Length of residency also tended to be associated characteristically with these several influences. Doctors for whom intellectual influences were important in selecting a practice field tended to report longer residency. This positive association was significant for both the public (CR 2.3) and private (CR 2.05) school graduates of 1954 but was not significant for those of 1950. The negative association between the influence of finances and the length of residency was significant for all groups (CR range from 2.1 to 3.6) except for the 1954 private school graduates. When social pressures were reported to be important these were also negatively associated with the length of residency. This negative association was significant only for the private school graduates (CR 2.4 for 1950 and 2.7 for 1954 graduates).

The doctors' responses about the various influences which determined their decision about a field of practice show a consistent and credible relation to the actual preparation they obtained for their careers. Intellectual interests were more frequently associated with internship in a teaching hospital, with a straight rather than a rotating internship, with some residency training rather than none, and with more prolonged residency training.

Conversely, as might be expected, influences such as finances, social pressures, and spouse were associated with choice of nonteaching hospitals and shorter training. Doctors who prepared for practice with a rotating internship in a minor or nonteaching hospital, and who obtained little or no residency training, exhibit a certain urgency to enter practice that is consistent with their reports of the factors—for example, finances—that influenced their choices.

It is, of course, important to recognize that these reports by doctors as to the factors that influenced their career choices are not only subjective but retrospective. It is possible, for example, that physicians who now regret the brevity of their training (or some other aspect of their choices) are reporting financial or other reasons as justification, when other factors may, in fact, have been influential at the time. Despite the limitations of subjective and retrospective reports, however, there are many reasons to believe that the reported factors were actually important. Especially convincing is the fact that these data are consistent with many other aspects of the doctors' responses—on working during medical school, on total debts, and the like.

It is also worthy of note that these reports by doctors about factors influencing their choices of field of practice are associated with class rank (Table 41). For example, physicians in the top third of their class reported the influence of intellectual interests significantly more frequently than those in the middle or lowest third except among private school graduates of 1954, among whom this trend was present but weak (CR 2.1 for 1950 and 4.8 for 1954 public school graduates; CR 1.9 for private school graduates in 1950). Those who stated that finances were a consideration more frequently ranked in the bottom third of their class. This effect is apparent mainly in the public schools, and even there it was not of large magnitude for the 1950 graduates. Regression analysis showed a strong significant association (CR

TABLE 41. Percent of doctors strongly influenced in choice of field of practice by influential factor, by class rank in thirds, type of school, and year of graduation

| Influential factor | Public | | | | | | Private | | | | | |
|---|---|---|---|---|---|---|---|---|---|---|---|---|
| | 1950 | | | 1954 | | | 1950 | | | 1954 | | |
| | Upper | Middle | Lower | Upper | Middle | Lower | Upper | Middle | Lower | Upper | Middle | Lower |
| Intellectual | 80 | 70 | 64 | 86 | 72 | 66 | 85 | 80 | 77 | 89 | 86 | 87 |
| Finances | 22 | 33 | 33 | 15 | 24 | 29 | 15 | 19 | 19 | 11 | 11 | 12 |
| | (111) | (120) | (103) | (156) | (194) | (148) | (149) | (144) | (137) | (175) | (170) | (164) |

3.5) between class rank and the influence of finances for the 1954 public school graduates. Social pressures, influence of spouse, and special patient interests showed no association with class rank.

The MCAT scores, which were available only for 1954 classes, showed no consistent relationships to the doctors' reports of factors which influenced their decisions about field of practice.

*Interrelationship of Training Variables*

It is clear that the factors influencing training are multiple and that none are clearly decisive with respect to such decisions as who will intern in a major teaching hospital or who will obtain some residency. Moreover, trainees are culled and selected at all stages of medical school internship, and residency. Before proceeding to an examination of the interrelationship of the various influential factors, it is important to review the major differences in the training of the private and public medical school graduates.

In Chapter IV the types of internships reported by the private and public school graduates were shown (Table 27). The high proportion (almost 90 percent) of the public school graduates who began training with a rotating internship contrasted with the much smaller proportion (just over 50 percent) of the private school graduates who reported this type of internship. Far more of the private school graduates reported major teaching hospital internships in both 1950 (CR 2.5) and 1954 (CR 2.4) (Table 29). The public school graduates were also very different in that they reported no residency far more frequently than did private school graduates; these differences were highly significant in both 1950 (CR 8.9) and 1954 (CR 5.0) (Table 30). The frequency of reported residency increased significantly for both public and private school graduates between 1950 and 1954. The critical ratio for the public school difference from 1950 to 1954 was 2.5; that for the corresponding private school increase was 4.1.

As Table 42 shows, physicians who interned in a major teaching hospital were more likely to proceed on into a residency training than those who interned in other institutions. This difference was significant for all groups except the 1954 public school graduate for whom the critical ratio was borderline (1.9); among the other groups the critical ratio values ranged from 2.8 to 9.4. Regardless of internship the public school graduates reported no residency with significantly greater frequency than did the private school groups: these differences were significant in both 1950 and 1954 (CR range 3.8 to 7.8). Internship in a major teaching hospital was also likely to be followed by a longer period of residency, when residency was obtained. This effect was more marked in 1950 than in 1954, and more striking in public than in private schools; in private schools, even among those who interned in hospitals other than major teaching, more than two thirds obtained at least two years of residency in the 1950 class and 82 percent did so in the 1954 class. The difference in frequency of longer residency (twenty-four months or more) among doctors who interned in major teaching and those who interned in other hospitals was significant for all groups except the public 1954 graduates. The critical ratio values ranged from 2.7 to 7.0 for the other three groups.

As Table 43 shows, the type of internship is significantly associated with residency experience. In both 1950 and 1954, and in both public and private schools, a straight internship (virtually all in major teaching hospitals) is almost always a prelude to a residency; a rotating internship in a major teaching hospital leads to residency less frequently, and a rotating internship in another hospital is least likely to lead to residency. Thus, the proportion

TABLE 42. Percentage distribution of doctors by hospital of internship, months of residency, type of school, and year of graduation

|  | Public | | | | Private | | | |
|---|---|---|---|---|---|---|---|---|
|  | 1950 | | 1954 | | 1950 | | 1954 | |
| Months of residency | Major teaching | Other | Major teaching | Other | Major teaching | Other | Major teaching | Other |
| None | 21 | 35 | 18 | 30 | 4 | 17 | 2 | 8 |
| 1 - 23 | 6 | 11 | 12 | 10 | 7 | 15 | 8 | 10 |
| 24 - 47 | 52 | 37 | 53 | 45 | 61 | 46 | 55 | 54 |
| 48 - | 21 | 18 | 18 | 16 | 28 | 22 | 35 | 28 |
|  | (132) | (199) | (210) | (285) | (278) | (149) | (354) | (154) |

TABLE 43. Percent of doctors reporting residency by type of internship, type of school, and year of graduation

| Type of internship | Public | | Private | |
|---|---|---|---|---|
| | 1950 | 1954 | 1950 | 1954 |
| All straight | 91 (23) | 95 (39) | 99 (162) | 99 (215) |
| Rotating in major teaching hospital | 73 (98) | 80 (168) | 93 (99) | 97 (123) |
| Rotating - other | 65 (192) | 70 (277) | 81 (135) | 91 (148) |

of physicians with straight internship (including obstetrics-gynecology, pediatrics, and other straight services) reporting a residency is significantly greater than the proportion of physicians with rotating internship reporting a residency in both public and private schools in 1950 (CR 3.8 and 2.6) and in public schools in 1954 (CR 3.3). The same pattern is evident when those with rotating internships are compared with those who chose straight medical or straight surgical internships.

When physicians who took rotating internships in a major teaching hospital are compared with those who took rotating internships in a nonteaching hospital, the former were significantly more likely to obtain residency in both public and private schools in 1950 (CR 2.8 and 4.1) and in private schools in 1954 (CR 2.3).

Among physicians who took rotating internships—whether in a major teaching hospital or in another hospital—the private school graduates were far more likely than public school graduates to take a residency in both 1950 and 1954 (CR range from 3.7 to 6.4). Among those who took straight internships, however, there was no such striking public-private school difference with regard to residency training, although the difference reached the borderline of significance (CR 1.9) when 1950 public and private school graduates with straight internships in a major teaching hospital were compared.

The differences in obtaining residency between physicians with straight and rotating internships, in major teaching hospitals or other hospitals, disappear when residency training of twenty-four months or longer duration is specified, and there are no significant differences by type of internship between public and private school graduates in this group.

*Academic Achievement and Training Variables*

An examination of the relationship between the Medical College Admissions Test composite score and medical school performance on the one hand and internship and residency on the other has been the subject of a previous publication.(22) Here we will deal with only the major associations.

There was, first of all, an apparent difference in the distributions of public and private school graduates by MCAT scores. As explained in Chapter IV, much of this public-private difference was due to the scores of the students in three private schools selected because a high proportion of their graduates had entered teaching or research careers. The distribution of scores in the other three private schools was quite similar to the majority of the public schools. One public school had an unusually high number of high scoring students; about a third scored above 600. Thus there is a considerable overlap in the distributions of students' scores in the two types of institutions. The differences between public and private schools shown in Table 44 are not significant.

TABLE 44. Percentage distribution of 1954 graduates by MCAT scores

|  | 601- | 501-600 | -500 | No record |
|---|---|---|---|---|
| Public | 17 | 48 | 26 | 9 (498) |
| Private | 39 | 40 | 16 | 5 (509) |

The Medical College Admission Test showed a variable association with the type of internship obtained. Among the public school graduates for whom MCAT scores were available, about 88 percent of those with scores below 500 reported a rotating internship, in contrast to 80 percent of the students whose MCAT scores were above 600. The private school graduates exhibited much greater diversity in selecting internships and the relationship to MCAT scores appeared to be more definite (Table 45). Regression analysis did not demonstrate that either of these associations was significant, however.

TABLE 45. Percentage distribution of doctors by type of internship, by composite MCAT score, 1954 graduates only, by type of school

| Type of internship | Public | | | Private | | |
|---|---|---|---|---|---|---|
|  | -500 | 501-600 | 601- | -500 | 501-600 | 601- |
| Rotating | 88 | 87 | 80 | 63 | 56 | 46 |
| Straight medical or surgical | 4 | 6 | 11 | 23 | 35 | 40 |
| Other | 0 | 2 | 2 | 8 | 6 | 10 |
| No response | 7 | 4 | 7 | 6 | 3 | 4 |
|  | (127) | (238) | (87) | (81) | (203) | (201) |

Straight internships in medicine or surgery showed an association opposite to the rotating training, as would be expected. This association was significant for the private school graduates (CR 2.06), but not for the public school group. Other types of internships, including mixed services and a small number of other straight services, show no specific associations.

The MCAT scores also seemed to have some relationship to the type of hospital in which internship was obtained (Table 46). Among the public school graduates this relationship is at best suggestive. Among the private school graduates, on the other hand, there is a clear linear relationship between the MCAT score and the hospital of internship, which proved to be significant (CR 2.2). Internship in minor teaching hospitals is inversely associated with MCAT scores. The resemblance of minor teaching hospitals and nonteaching hospitals is illustrated in

TABLE 46. Percent of doctors by hospital of internship by composite MCAT score, 1954 graduates only, by type of school

| Hospital of internship | Public | | | Private | | |
|---|---|---|---|---|---|---|
| | -500 | 501-600 | 601- | -500 | 501-600 | 601- |
| Major teaching | 36 | 41 | 40 | 48 | 64 | 78 |
| Minor teaching | 17 | 12 | 10 | 12 | 8 | 2 |
| Non-teaching approved | 39 | 44 | 45 | 37 | 25 | 17 |
| Other | 0 | 0 | 1 | 0 | 0 | 0 |
| No response | 7 | 3 | 4 | 2 | 3 | 3 |
| | (127) | (238) | (87) | (81) | (203) | (201) |

Table 46. In the case of private school graduates, nonteaching approved internships attract a larger proportion of men with low than with high MCAT scores, but this was not clearly the case with the public school group. (Since the characteristics of doctors reporting minor teaching hospital internships closely resemble those of doctors with nonteaching hospital experience, the two groups have been combined in most of the following tables.)

MCAT results also appear to bear a variable relationship to reported residency training (Table 47). The negative relationship between MCAT scores and the frequency of no residency shown by the public school graduates was significant (CR 2.5) but the similar trend shown by the private school groups was not.

TABLE 47. Percent of doctors with no residency by MCAT score, 1954 graduates, by type of school

|  | Public | | | Private | | |
|---|---|---|---|---|---|---|
|  | -500 | 501-600 | 601- | -500 | 501-600 | 601- |
| No residency | 35 | 18 | 20 | 7 | 3 | 4 |
|  | (127) | (238) | (87) | (81) | (203) | (201) |

The selection of a major teaching hospital residency was examined in relation to MCAT scores. Although higher scores seemed to be regularly associated with major teaching hospital residency, regression analysis failed to show significance either for public or private school graduates. The length of residency did not vary in any systematic fashion with the MCAT score.

Gough and his coworkers, who have extensively reviewed medical school admissions procedures, state: "The MCAT appears to have at best a low validity for forecasting performance in school and for completion of training. With respect to each criteria of performance in internship and professional practice, the validity is essentially zero."(12) Among the schools in our sample the test was a poor predictor of performance in medical school.(24) The science section correlated with class rank sufficiently to reach significance in about half of the classes. The remainder of the test and the composite score showed less relationship with rank. It is not surprising to find that the composite score, which was a very poor forecaster of academic performance, shows few regular associations with the internship and residency.

Other workers have found the same low correlation between MCAT scores and medical school grades that is reported here. Any predictive value of the MCAT with respect to the internship and residency does not seem to have been examined previously. It may be that, with more detailed analysis, the test will prove to be useful as an indicator of training potential rather than of success in medical school.(4) Its predictive value may also be greater within smaller groups of schools.

As one might suspect, rank in medical school class has a relation to the hospital chosen and the type of internship. All groups showed a negative association between class rank and the frequency of reported rotating internships (see Table 48). In the case of the public school graduates this association was regular but neither strong nor significant. The association was stronger for the private school graduates; by regression analysis it was found to be definitely significant for the 1950 private school classes (CR 2.4) and borderline for the 1954 private school classes (CR 1.9). The positive association between class rank and reporting of straight medical internships was significant for all groups except the 1950 public school graduates; the small number of doctors (twelve) in this group who reported straight

TABLE 48. Percent of doctors by class rank with rotating or straight medical internship by type of school and year of graduation

|  | Public | | | Private | | |
|---|---|---|---|---|---|---|
|  | Lower | Middle | Upper | Lower | Middle | Upper |
|  | | | 1950 | | | |
| Rotating | 94 | 91 | 85 | 72 | 54 | 42 |
| Straight medical | 1 | 3 | 8 | 12 | 16 | 36 |
|  | (101) | (115) | (107) | (136) | (140) | (145) |
|  | | | 1954 | | | |
| Rotating | 98 | 92 | 84 | 65 | 57 | 40 |
| Straight medical | 1 | 5 | 12 | 12 | 17 | 35 |
|  | (149) | (188) | (153) | (162) | (168) | (171) |

medical internships probably explains this nonsignificance. Among the other three groups the critical ratios ranged from 2.1 to 2.7. The men with straight surgical training, as well as "other" internships, were drawn from all ranks without any evident suggestion of special selection. This is consistent with material presented in Chapter IV which indicated that internists were drawn disproportionately from the higher ranked students whereas surgeons did not show any such relationship.

The differences between public and private schools described above are given further support when the hospital of internship is examined in relation to class rank. Here class rank exercises its influence upon graduates of both groups of schools (Table 49).

It will be recalled that more of the private school graduates reported major teaching hospital internships and that this difference between public and private schools was significant for both

TABLE 49. Percent of doctors reporting major teaching hospital internship by class rank and by type of school

|  | Public | | | Private | | |
|---|---|---|---|---|---|---|
|  | Lower | Middle | Upper | Lower | Middle | Upper |
| 1950 | 31 (103) | 37 (119) | 52 (109) | 50 (136) | 67 (144) | 78 (147) |
| 1954 | 25 (147) | 46 (194) | 54 (154) | 57 (164) | 69 (170) | 82 (174) |

1950 and 1954 graduates. It is clear from Table 49 that major teaching hospital internships also are associated with class rank for both public and private school graduates. These associations were found to be significant by regression analysis except in the case of the 1954 private school graduates (CR 1.6). The critical ratio values for the other groups were as follows: public, 1950, CR 3.09; private, 1950, CR 2.1; and public, 1954, CR 3.2. The minor teaching hospitals resembled the nonteaching hospitals in that they attracted more graduates who ranked in the bottom third of their class and fewer who ranked in the upper third.

Class rank was also positively associated with residency training (Table 50). This association was manifestly weak in the case

TABLE 50. Percent of doctors with residency training by class rank and type of school

|  | Public | | | Private | | |
|---|---|---|---|---|---|---|
|  | Lower | Middle | Upper | Lower | Middle | Upper |
| 1950 | 68 (103) | 66 (120) | 77 (111) | 89 (137) | 90 (144) | 95 (149) |
| 1954 | 67 (148) | 72 (194) | 87 (156) | 93 (164) | 96 (170) | 98 (175) |

of the 1950 public school graduates and its significance proved to be borderline (CR about 1.9). Among the other three groups the associations were consistent and definitely significant when the trend was tested. The critical ratio values were: 2.5 for the 1950 private school graduates; 3.6 for the 1954 public, and 8.6 for the 1954 private school graduates.

The attainment of residency in a major teaching hospital may also be associated with medical school performance. Except for the 1950 public school graduates, who showed no trend, higher class rank was associated more frequently with major teaching hospital residency than was lower rank. Although the trends shown by the other three groups were consistent, the only one that was significant was that for the 1954 private school graduates (CR 2.3). In this last group the percents of doctors whose residency was in a major teaching hospital varied from 36 percent in the lowest third of their class to 42 percent in the middle and 63 percent in the upper third.

*Family Background*

Analysis of variance indicated that the small differences in the family backgrounds of the 1950 or 1954 graduates of public and private medical schools as measured by the educational level of fathers were usually not significant. As illustrated in Table 51, the education of fathers of private school graduates as compared with those of public school graduates was somewhat less frequently limited to grade or high school and more frequently included some postcollege experience. The difference between private and public schools in reported frequency of fathers with some postgraduate education in 1954 was the only one that was significant (CR 2.6).

TABLE 51. Percentage distribution of doctors by father's education

|  | Public | | Private | |
|---|---|---|---|---|
|  | 1950 | 1954 | 1950 | 1954 |
| No college | 55 | 54 | 51 | 42 |
| Some college | 21 | 26 | 23 | 25 |
| Postgraduate | 24 | 21 | 27 | 32 |
|  | (324) | (492) | (423) | (502) |

When father's education is examined in relation to the doctors' training and ability, it appears to have a variable association. It shows no relationship with the Medical College Admission Test or with class rank in medical school. The failure of these conventional means of appraising medical students' ability to discriminate between students of diverse backgrounds suggest that the applicants' competence is the major determinant of admission and is independent of other student or family characteristics. This is not a surprising conclusion, but it is emphasized here because medical students are chosen from the population in a very skewed fashion, as was shown in a preceding chapter.

Father's education did not show any association with the type of internship obtained by these doctors, that is, it did not appear to be related to the choice of a rotating or straight internship. It did, however, show some association with the hospital of internship, for public and private school graduates of 1950 and 1954 (Table 52). In each of these groups the doctors who interned in major teaching hospitals had fewer fathers whose education was high school or less and more fathers with college or postgraduate education than did those who interned in other hospitals. The

TABLE 52. Percentage distribution of doctors by father's education, hospital of internship, type of school, and year of graduation

| Father's education | Public | | | | Private | | | |
|---|---|---|---|---|---|---|---|---|
| | 1950 | | 1954 | | 1950 | | 1954 | |
| | Major teaching | Other | Major teaching | Other | Major teaching | Other | Major teaching | Other |
| No college | 51 | 58 | 48 | 58 | 47 | 58 | 37 | 55 |
| College | 49 | 42 | 52 | 42 | 53 | 42 | 63 | 45 |
| | (127) | (194) | (208) | (282) | (274) | (146) | (352) | (149) |

small difference for the 1950 public school graduates is not significant. The differences for the other three groups were all significant (CR range from 2.1 to 3.1).

A similar though less definite association was evident with residency training (Table 53). In all groups the doctors who trained in major teaching hospitals seemingly were less likely to have fathers with limited education and more likely to have fathers with college or postgraduate education. None of these findings with respect to differences in residencies was significant.

A somewhat larger proportion of doctors without than with residency training reported that their fathers had a high school or less education. No residency was also associated with fewer fathers with some college education or postgraduate study. However, none of these differences was significant. The length of residency did not show a strong association with father's education.

When mother's education was examined, somewhat similar though even weaker associations were found. Since marriage is usually a union of like with like, this is not unexpected. Rather few of the doctors (3–7 percent) in various groups reported that their mothers had obtained any postgraduate education, so the comparison is largely limited to those with high school and college educations.

Mother's education showed no relationship with MCAT scores or class rank in medical school. It was associated with hospital of internship in a way quite similar to father's education; doctors who interned in major teaching hospitals had mothers with more college education than those trained in other institutions. More maternal education was associated with major teaching hospital residencies in the case of all public school graduates and the private 1950 graduates. There was no association with the "residency" and "no residency" groups. Thus, the

TABLE 53. Percentage distribution of doctors by father's education and by hospital of residency, by type of school, and by year of graduation

| Father's education | Public | | | | Private | | | |
|---|---|---|---|---|---|---|---|---|
| | 1950 | | 1954 | | 1950 | | 1954 | |
| | Major teaching | Other | Major teaching | Other | Major teaching | Other | Major teaching | Other |
| No College | 45 | 59 | 47 | 55 | 44 | 53 | 41 | 42 |
| College 1-4 years | 21 | 18 | 28 | 24 | 22 | 23 | 26 | 25 |
| College over 4 years | 31 | 21 | 25 | 19 | 33 | 23 | 33 | 30 |
| No response | 3 | 2 | 1 | 1 | 1 | 1 | 1 | 2 |
| | (80) | (154) | (159) | (215) | (170) | (222) | (234) | (255) |

mother's education showed some of the associations with doctors' training that were found in the case of fathers. The reason for these associations can only be speculative. It was evident, however, that the association is more consistently related to the father's than to the mother's educational history. None of the associations between mother's education and the several training variables being considered were definite enough to merit testing for significance.

The doctors' ethnic background as judged by their fathers' country of origin generally had no consistent effect upon or association with any aspect of medical education or training with one exception, already mentioned in Chapter IV: doctors whose fathers were of Eastern European and Eastern Mediterranean origin consistently ranked higher in their medical school classes than doctors with other ethnic backgrounds, who showed no consistent tendency to rank either high or low. The variation exhibited by this group (Table 54) is emphasized by the fact that class rank of all doctors describes approximate thirds of each group. The tendency of the doctors with Eastern European and

TABLE 54. Percentage distribution of doctors of Eastern European and Eastern Mediterranean background by class rank, by type of school, and by year of graduation

|  | Public | | Private | |
|---|---|---|---|---|
|  | 1950 | 1954 | 1950 | 1954 |
| Upper | 48 | 43 | 43 | 44 |
| Middle | 30 | 34 | 33 | 31 |
| Lower | 23 | 23 | 23 | 25 |
|  | (44) | (61) | (69) | (89) |

Eastern Mediterranean backgrounds to rank high in their classes was significant for each group. The critical ratios were as follows: public school graduates of 1950, 4.8; private, 1950, 3.5; public, 1954, 6.4; and private, 1954, 3.12. This group was not consistently different from all others with respect to the MCAT scores.

The doctors with this ethnic background reported residency training more frequently than all doctors, and their residencies tended to be longer. The private school graduates of Eastern European and East Mediterranean backgrounds reported some residency training significantly more frequently than fellow graduates with other backgrounds in both 1950 (CR 2.1) and 1954 (CR 2.7). Although the public school graduates in this group also reported more frequent residencies than their classmates, these differences were not significant either for the 1950 or 1954 classes. However, the tendency to take long residency was not completely consistent and cannot be regarded as more than suggestive. A small group of doctors with other ethnic backgrounds also tended to be outstanding in terms of academic performance and training. It was extremely heterogeneous and included doctors of various Asian backgrounds, Negroes, and South Americans. It was both too small and too diverse to be suitable for comparisons. This group was obviously highly selected.

Doctors with mothers whose origin was Eastern European or Eastern Mediterranean showed tendencies similar to those reported above. The doctors in this group reported no residency about half as frequently as the generality of doctors, and also tended to rank somewhat higher in their classes. Thus it appears that ethnic background has little influence on or relation with performance in medical school or training obtained thereafter, with the possible exception of doctors with fathers (and mothers) whose origins were in Eastern Europe or the Eastern Mediterranean area.

It will be recalled that the doctors included in this study were drawn from very diverse family backgrounds as judged from their fathers' occupations. The many different occupations followed by the fathers of these doctors are obviously associated with differences in education and income, which, in turn, might influence or limit a doctor's education or training for practice. As illustrated in the previous chapter, there were no important differences in the distribution of reported occupations of fathers of public and private school graduates, nor was there any clear change between 1950 and 1954. The single exception was the greater proportion of doctors' sons among the 1954 private school graduates when compared with the public school group; this difference was significant (CR 3.2).

Father's occupation did not appear to influence doctors in their choice of a rotating or straight internship. It did appear to be related to the hospital of internship for the group of doctors whose fathers were craftsmen. From Table 55 it can be seen that this group interned in major teaching hospitals in a smaller proportion of instances than all other doctors and, conversely, interned more often in the other institutions. The "craftsmen" classification includes a variety of blue collar occupations including skilled and unskilled labor. It is the occupational group with the lowest average income and least education. The difference between craftsmen's sons and other doctors was significant only for the 1950 public school graduates (CR 2.1).

The possible different influences of private and public schools or possible differences in the type of students they obtain is also reflected in Table 55. A higher proportion of craftsmen's sons who graduated from private schools reported major teaching hos-

TABLE 55. Percentage distribution of doctors by father's occupation and by hospital of internship, sons of craftsmen and all others, and by type of school and year of graduation

| Father's occupation | Public | | | | Private | | | |
|---|---|---|---|---|---|---|---|---|
| | 1950 | | 1954 | | 1950 | | 1954 | |
| | Major teaching | Other | Major teaching | Other | Major teaching | Other | Major teaching | Other |
| Craftsmen | 27 | 73 ( 56) | 34 | 66 ( 97) | 47 | 53 ( 76) | 52 | 48 ( 85) |
| All others | 42 | 58 (269) | 44 | 56 (392) | 70 | 30 (343) | 74 | 26 (308) |

pital internships than did the same group who graduated from public schools. These differences however, were not significant in either 1950 or 1954. The proportion of craftsmen's sons in each group varied little between private and public schools or between 1950 and 1954 (range, 17–19 percent).

The proportion of doctors reporting residency training in major teaching hospitals increased for all doctors for both public and private schools between 1950 and 1954. The proportion of sons of craftsmen with major teaching hospital residencies increased somewhat more rapidly than the proportion of all doctors. With the exception of the 1954 public school graduates, where craftsmen's sons did not differ from the whole group, they showed the same association with residency training that was found for the internship—that is, the proportion with major teaching hospital residency is less than for all doctors (Table 56).

The proportion of graduates who did not obtain residency training is strongly influenced by the type of medical school (public or private), but very little by father's occupation (Table 57). For each occupational group the public school graduates reported no residency more frequently than did the private school groups. Table 57 shows there is no consistent association between father's occupation and the frequency of no residency training, although in two of the four groups doctors' sons had the smallest proportion with no residency.

When length of residency is examined, by father's occupation, only one group stands out, and not markedly: in three of the four groups the percent of doctors' sons with the longest training exceeded all others and in the 1950 private school group they were equaled only by sons of executives. When the doctors' sons were compared with all other respondents with respect to very

TABLE 56. Percentage distribution of doctors by father's occupation and by hospital of residency, sons of craftsmen and all others, and by type of school and year of graduation

| Father's occupation | Public | | | | Private | | | |
|---|---|---|---|---|---|---|---|---|
| | 1950 | | 1954 | | 1950 | | 1954 | |
| | Major teaching | Other | Major teaching | Other | Major teaching | Other | Major teaching | Other |
| Craftsmen | 23 | 77 ( 39) | 42 | 58 ( 67) | 29 | 71 ( 70) | 43 | 57 ( 82) |
| All others | 37 | 63 (190) | 42 | 58 (303) | 47 | 53 (317) | 50 | 50 (400) |

TABLE 57. Percentage distribution of doctors by father's occupation, by no residency and by months of residency, type of school, and year of graduation

|  | 1950 | | | 1954 | | |
|---|---|---|---|---|---|---|
|  | None | 1-47 | 48- | None | 1-47 | 48- |
| | Public | | | | | |
| Physician | 22 | 46 | 32 (37) | 12 | 50 | 38 (50) |
| Executive | 28 | 48 | 24 (25) | 7 | 75 | 18 (44) |
| Craftsmen | 30 | 46 | 23 (56) | 31 | 59 | 10 (97) |
| Other | 41 | 37 | 22 (27) | 37 | 51 | 11 (35) |
| Semi-professional/clerical | 34 | 49 | 17 (53) | 33 | 59 | 8 (66) |
| Small business | 27 | 57 | 16 (67) | 21 | 59 | 20 (113) |
| Professional | 32 | 59 | 10 (63) | 27 | 58 | 15 (86) |
| | Private | | | | | |
| Physician | 3 | 65 | 32 (60) | 5 | 51 | 45 (85) |
| Executive | 10 | 58 | 32 (40) | 6 | 59 | 35 (66) |
| Craftsmen | 8 | 66 | 26 (76) | 4 | 74 | 22 (85) |
| Other | 14 | 62 | 24 (21) | 16 | 53 | 32 (19) |
| Semi-professional/clerical | 10 | 68 | 22 (69) | 3 | 64 | 32 (74) |
| Small business | 8 | 70 | 22 (87) | 3 | 70 | 28 (79) |
| Professional | 7 | 67 | 26 (69) | 3 | 61 | 36 (94) |

long residencies (forty-eight months or more) differences were significant for all groups except the 1950 private school graduates. The critical ratio values for the differences between doctors' sons and all others were 2.6 for the public 1950 classes, 3.3 for the public 1954 classes, and 2.6 for the private 1954 classes. Craftsmen's sons are not different from other doctors by this measure.

*Place of Birth*

This examination of place of birth will attempt to see what association birth in a large city, suburban area, or small city or town may have with doctor's preparation for practice.

The MCAT scores show little association with birthplace and none that was significant. Doctors born in small towns tended to be underrepresented in the highest MCAT group whereas those born in large cities were overrepresented. Doctors born elsewhere (that is, in suburbs or small cities) did not differ consistently from all doctors for whom MCAT scores were available.

There was a similar relationship with class rank: only doctors born in small towns and large cities were different and only in the 1954 classes (Table 58). Doctors who were born in small

TABLE 58. Percentage distribution of doctors born in large cities or in small towns by class rank, 1954 graduates only, by type of school

|  | Public | | | Private | | |
| --- | --- | --- | --- | --- | --- | --- |
|  | Upper | Middle | Lower | Upper | Middle | Lower |
| Small town | 27 | 35 | 38 (149) | 21 | 37 | 43 ( 82) |
| Large city | 37 | 40 | 33 (187) | 40 | 33 | 27 (256) |

towns (population less than ten thousand) were overrepresented in the lowest third of their classes in both the public (CR 4.9) and private (CR 4.4) school groups graduating in 1954. Large-city origin is definitely associated with higher class rank for the private school graduates of 1954 (CR 4.2), but there is no definite association in the other groups. Although these trends are significant, the failure to find similar associations for 1950 graduates or to find them consistently present for 1954 makes it difficult to evaluate their importance.

Place of birth showed no association with type of internship or the hospital of internship. Similarly, the hospital and length of residency did not vary in any consistent manner with place of birth. Doctors who reported medical residencies were born in cities of population over 50,000 with somewhat greater frequency than all doctors. Though these differences were not great, they were consistent and were present in each group. Doctors reporting psychiatric residencies exhibited consistently greater frequency of large-city birth. Whereas 43 percent of all doctors were born in large cities (population over 100,000), 64 percent of those with psychiatric residencies were born there. This was true for both public and private school graduates of 1950 and 1954 (Table 59).

*Age at Graduation*

Age at graduation might be expected to affect training in a number of ways. Students may be older because they are less able and experienced difficulty in obtaining admission to medical school. Older graduates may be impatient for a good income and shorten their training. Financial problems may interrupt an education or delay its completion. The possibilities of being married

TABLE 59. Percentage distribution of doctors reporting psychiatric residency and all others by place of birth

| Birthplace | Psychiatric residency | All other |
|---|---|---|
| Small town | 17 | 24 |
| Medium city | 12 | 21 |
| Large city | 64 | 43 |
| Suburbs | 4 | 6 |
| Other | 3 | 5 |
|  | (114) | (1657) |

increase with age, and pressures upon the doctor from spouse or family might also increase.

There were differences between the public and private school graduates in our sample by age at graduation, as illustrated in Table 20. The extent to which training has any association with public or private medical school educations, per se, may be affected by the greater proportion of younger graduates of the private schools.

The MCAT scores, which bear some relationship to ability, do not provide any positive evidence of an age relationship. There was a slight suggestion that greater age at graduation was associated with a lower score and younger age with higher score.

By contrast the association between class rank and age was definite. In every group a higher proportion of the older graduates was found in this lowest rank than was the case of the younger graduates, who were concentrated to a greater degree in the top rank (Table 60). Testing of the negative association

TABLE 60. Percentage distribution of doctors by age at graduation and class rank, by type of school and year of graduation

| Age | 1950 Public | | | 1950 Private | | | 1954 Public | | | 1954 Private | | |
|---|---|---|---|---|---|---|---|---|---|---|---|---|
| | Upper | Middle | Lower | Upper | Middle | Lower | Upper | Middle | Lower | Upper | Middle | Lower |
| 29- | 40 | 48 | 53 | 33 | 34 | 44 | 10 | 26 | 28 | 7 | 8 | 18 |
| 27-28 | 19 | 21 | 17 | 16 | 26 | 15 | 22 | 29 | 30 | 20 | 26 | 31 |
| -26 | 41 | 32 | 29 | 50 | 35 | 36 | 65 | 44 | 40 | 72 | 64 | 48 |
| N.R. | 1 | 0 | 1 | 1 | 4 | 5 | 3 | 1 | 1 | 1 | 2 | 3 |
| | (111) | (120) | (103) | (149) | (144) | (137) | (156) | (194) | (148) | (175) | (170) | (164) |

between greater age (defined as age of twenty-nine or more years) and class rank showed that it was significant for the 1950 public school graduates (CR 2.1) but not for the private school graduates of that year. Among the 1954 graduates the association was significant; the critical ratio for the trend shown by the public school graduates was 4.1 and for the private school graduates, 3.8. Among the younger graduates—age twenty-six or less—the tendency to rank high in the class was not significant among either public or private graduates of 1950. In 1954 the trend was significant, however, for both the public (CR 4.1) and private school graduates (CR 2.7). Other studies have shown that failure rates in medical school are higher among the older students. Thus attrition presumably thinned the ranks of the older doctors in this study more severely than the younger. Nevertheless the negative association between greater age and class rank is still apparent. The effect was much more marked in 1954 than in 1950. This may be related to the fact that many of the older students in the 1950 class were returning veterans, who were an unusual group academically. (9, 15, 16, 27)

The type of internship, whether rotating or other, did not show any association with doctors' ages at graduation. The hospital of internship did (Table 61). Doctors who were twenty-nine or older at the time of graduation interned less often in major teaching hospitals and more frequently in other hospitals. When this age group is compared with younger doctors (age twenty-eight or less) the results are significant (CR range from 2.9 to 4.4) for all groups except the public school 1954 graduates, for whom the critical ratio value for the difference is borderline (1.9). The youngest group of doctors—twenty-six years or less—reported major teaching hospital internships more frequently than all other doctors; the differences between this

TABLE 61. Percentage distribution of doctors by age at graduation and hospital of internship

| Age | 1950 ||||| 1954 |||||
| | Public || Private || Public || Private ||
| | Major teaching | Other | Major teaching | Other | Major teaching | Other | Major teaching | Other |
|---|---|---|---|---|---|---|---|---|
| 29- | 38 | 53 | 32 | 46 | 17 | 25 | 8 | 18 |
| 27-28 | 19 | 18 | 18 | 21 | 28 | 28 | 23 | 33 |
| -26 | 43 | 28 | 47 | 28 | 54 | 46 | 68 | 46 |
| No response | 0 | 1 | 2 | 6 | 2 | 1 | 2 | 3 |
| | (132) | (199) | (278) | (149) | (210) | (285) | (254) | (154) |

youngest group and all other doctors were not significant for the 1954 public school graduates, but were for all other groups (CR range from 2.3 to 3.8). It should be noted that between 1950 and 1954 there was an increase in the proportion of internships served in major teaching hospitals. This is presumably related to the increase in the number of these more desirable training positions.

Residency training is also strongly influenced by or related to age at graduation (Table 62). In comparison with all doctors, those who reported no residency tended to be older. The doctors who were age twenty-nine or greater at the time of graduation reported no residency with significantly greater frequency than their younger classmates. The critical ratio values for these differences were 3.1 and 4.6 for the public school graduates of 1950 and 1954 and 2.3 and 3.9 for the private school graduates of these years. There were, furthermore, important differences between public and private schools. The oldest public school graduates (age twenty-nine or greater) reported no residency significantly more frequently in 1950 (CR 6.3) and in 1954 (CR 4.4). The younger public school graduates (twenty-eight or less) also reported no residency more frequently than the younger private school graduates. This difference was significant in both 1950 (CR 3.7) and in 1954 (CR 4.6).

The hospital of residency showed some suggestive associations with doctors' ages at graduation. In most instances, the doctors who obtained all their residency in major teaching hospitals were drawn from the youngest graduates whereas the oldest graduates trained more frequently in other hospitals. Because of lack of consistency, this cannot be regarded as a definite association.

Men with surgical residency tended to be younger at graduation than all doctors in each group. Doctors who took medical

TABLE 62. Percentage distribution of doctors with residency and doctors with no residency by age at graduation, type of school, and year of graduation

|  | 1950 | | | | 1954 | | | |
|---|---|---|---|---|---|---|---|---|
|  | Public | | Private | | Public | | Private | |
| Age | Residency | No residency | Residency | No residency | Residency | No residency | Residency | No residency |
| 29- | 41 | 61 | 35 | 51 | 18 | 33 | 10 | 43 |
| 27-28 | 19 | 19 | 20 | 14 | 26 | 32 | 26 | 19 |
| -26 | 40 | 20 | 42 | 27 | 54 | 35 | 62 | 33 |
| No response | 1 | 0 | 3 | 8 | 2 | 1 | 2 | 5 |
|  | (234) | (100) | (393) | (37) | (375) | (123) | (488) | (21) |

residencies were the only other group represented with sufficient frequency to allow a detailed analysis. There was no consistent relationship between medical residency and age.

Among those doctors who reported residency training, its length did not correlate with the doctor's age.

*Sources of Support of Medical Students*

In the previous chapter the sources of support during medical education reported by the respondents were shown in three tables (21, 22, and 23). We have seen that general practitioners appeared to have had the most serious financial problems in obtaining a medical education since they reported more self-support and less parental support than other doctors. The possible effects of financial difficulties will be examined here in relation to academic performance and to internship and residency training.

In this study MCAT scores have shown little or no relationship with the family backgrounds of students. When these scores are examined in relation to the students' major source of support, rather few associations are found. In those instances where parents, a spouse, or loans were the major support there was no suggestion of any relationship. The most pronounced association was found among the 1954 private school graduates who received G.I. Bill support: among the students in these classes who ranked high, 15 percent received G.I. Bill support; the percentages were 20 and 35 for medium and low rank respectively. Regression analysis demonstrated that this association was at the borderline of significance (CR 1.98). A somewhat similar trend observed in the public school graduates was not significant. Among the doctors reporting other sources of support, there were no associations sufficiently definite to merit tests. Class rank did not in any way systematically reflect the source of student financial support. This finding again suggests that medical students are quite homogeneous in ability (as appraised by these measures), despite the extremely variable backgrounds from which they come.

Scholarships were an infrequent source of support and were only rarely a major source. Six percent of the public school graduates of 1950 reported some scholarship aid: this increased to about 15 percent among the public school respondents who graduated in 1954. The corresponding percents for the private school graduates were 17 percent in 1950 and 24 percent in 1954. The difference between public and private schools in frequency of reported scholarships was significant in 1950 (CR 2.2) but not in 1954. The increase in frequency of scholarships from 1950 to 1954 was not significant for either the public or private school graduates.

Among doctors who reported scholarships there were strong relationships to both MCAT scores and to class rank. Among the men with the highest MCAT score, more than twice as many reported scholarship aid as did the group with scores in the lowest category. Testing of this trend showed that it was significant for both the public (CR 2.5) and private school graduates (CR 3.4). Although the association between class rank and reported scholarships was suggestive for each group, it was significant for only one, the 1950 private school graduates (CR 2.2).

The student's source of support was related to the type of internship reported. Doctors who reported that the G.I. program or their spouse was a major source of support did not show a consistent pattern in their choice of an internship. Self and parental support, however, were associated with differences in the types of internships reported, as is shown in Table 63. Among public school graduates a higher proportion of those with

TABLE 63. Percent of doctors by rotating or straight medical or surgical internships by major source of support, type of school, and year of graduation

|  | Public | | Private | |
|---|---|---|---|---|
|  | 1950 | 1954 | 1950 | 1954 |
|  | Self-support | | | |
| Rotating | 13 (290) | 14 (446) | 4 (234) | 6 (271) |
| Straight | 5 (21) | 0 (37) | 4 (142) | 4 (184) |
|  | Parental support | | | |
| Rotating | 18 (290) | 30 (446) | 29 (234) | 47 (271) |
| Straight | 29 (21) | 54 (37) | 30 (142) | 57 (184) |

rotating than with straight medical or surgical internships reported self-support; the difference was significant for both the 1950 (CR 3.3) and 1954 graduates (CR 13). The private school graduates' choice of a rotating or straight internship was not related to self-support. Material presented in the preceding chapter demonstrated that the proportion of public school graduates who reported self-support was significantly greater than the proportion of the private school graduates. The selection of a rotating or a straight medical or surgical internship was somewhat different for the students whose major support was by parents. In general, the group who had straight internships reported parental support more frequently than doctors who had rotating internships. This difference was significant only for the public 1954 graduates (CR 2.0).

Internship in a major teaching hospital, in contrast with other hospital training, was associated with more parental support.

These differences were all significant (CR range from 2.5 to 3.7) except for the 1950 private school graduates. Major support by a spouse or self seemed to have no relation. Internship in other hospitals was consistently associated with more G.I. Bill support, but the differences were very small (Table 64).

Longer residency appeared to be associated with greater probability of parental support for public school graduates of 1950 and 1954, as is illustrated in Table 65. Doctors in these two groups who were supported by their parents reported no residency about half as frequently as other doctors. These differences were significant for 1950 (CR 3.0) and 1954 (CR 3.7). The differences reported by the private school graduates did not reach significance in either 1950 or 1954; the number in these cohorts with no residency training was very small and not significant despite the large difference in proportions. There is no difference in the frequency of residency training of intermediate length (one to twenty-three months.) The difference between doctors reporting major parental support and all others with respect to residency of twenty-four months or more was significant in both 1950 (CR 3.0) and 1954 (CR 3.7) for public school graduates. The same trends are apparent for the private school classes, but the differences are very small.

Two observations can be drawn from this tabulation. First, lack of major parental support appears to have a limiting effect upon residency training, and second, this effect is different for public and private school graduates. Where the spouse was a source of support, this appeared to be associated with shorter training.

The hospital in which residency was served apparently was associated with the type of student support in much the same manner as was the hospital of internship (Table 66). Parental

TABLE 64. Percent of all doctors with major teaching hospital or other internships by major source of support, type of school, and year of graduation

| | 1950 | | | | 1954 | | | |
| --- | --- | --- | --- | --- | --- | --- | --- | --- |
| | Public | | Private | | Public | | Private | |
| Major source | Major teaching | Other | Major teaching | Other | Major teaching | Other | Major teaching | Other |
| G.I. Bill | 20 | 30 | 21 | 23 | 4 | 8 | 1 | 4 |
| Parents | 27 | 15 | 31 | 25 | 44 | 24 | 54 | 44 |
| Self | 11 | 14 | 5 | 5 | 10 | 16 | 4 | 8 |
| Spouse | 7 | 5 | 5 | 5 | 5 | 9 | 4 | 3 |
| | (132) | (199) | (278) | (149) | (210) | (285) | (354) | (154) |

TABLE 65. Percentage distribution of doctors reporting major support by parents and all others by months of residency, by type of school, and by year of graduation

|  | Public | | | | | | | Private | | | |
|---|---|---|---|---|---|---|---|---|---|---|---|
|  | 1950 | | 1954 | | | 1950 | | | 1954 | | |
|  | Parental support | All other | Parental support | All other | | Parental support | All other | | Parental support | All other | |
| None | 14 | 34 | 13 | 30 | | 6 | 10 | | 2 | 6 | |
| 1-23 | 8 | 9 | 9 | 11 | | 11 | 9 | | 6 | 11 | |
| 24- | 79 | 57 | 78 | 58 | | 83 | 81 | | 92 | 83 | |
|  | (66) | (268) | (159) | (339) | | (123) | (307) | | (259) | (250) | |

TABLE 66. Percent of all doctors with major teaching and other hospital residency by major source of support, type of school, and year of graduation

| Major sources | 1950 | | | | 1954 | | | |
|---|---|---|---|---|---|---|---|---|
| | Public | | Private | | Public | | Private | |
| | Major teaching | Other | Major teaching | Other | Major teaching | Other | Major teaching | Other |
| G.I. Bill | 21 | 27 | 18 | 24 | 4 | 8 | 0 | 3 |
| Parents | 28 | 23 | 34 | 27 | 45 | 31 | 54 | 49 |
| | (80) | (154) | (170) | (222) | (159) | (215) | (234) | (255) |

support was more frequently reported by doctors who trained in major teaching hospitals whereas support from the G.I. Bill was more often a major source of support when residency was in the "other" group. Though these associations were consistent, they were not marked and cannot be regarded as more than suggestive.

Medical students are selected overwhelmingly from above-average income families. A recent study showed that nearly half had families with incomes above $10,000.(6) Where parental support is substantial, it is logical that it would permit additional training in preparation for practice; high or low levels of parental support might, furthermore, be important to decisions about training in major teaching hospitals (where renumeration is low) or in other institutions (where renumeration is greater). Where students support themselves or are supported by spouse or by loans, less training might be expected—and this is the case.

In the following pages, students have been divided into three groups according to their yearly earnings while in medical school: one group which comprises those who reported minimal or no yearly earnings (0–$499), a second intermediate group, and a third which includes those with high earnings ($1500 or more).

We have seen that the public and private school graduates reported different levels of earnings while they were in medical school (Table 24). In both 1950 and 1954 more public school graduates reported high earnings. Conversely, more of the private school graduates reported minimal yearly earnings. General practitioners, it will be recalled, were quite different from all doctors in that they more frequently reported high earnings while in medical school; since general practitioners are more frequently public school graduates, they account for much of the overall difference between public and private schools in this respect.

Doctors who reported high or low earnings were not clearly different with respect to ability as appraised by either the MCAT or class standing; however, there were differences between these two groups in respect to preparations for practice.

Greater annual earnings were more frequently associated with a rotating than a straight internship. Though this trend was consistent, it was, in general, not marked and reached a significant level only for the private school graduates of 1950 (CR 2.2). (See Table 67.) The hospital of internship also tended to be related to reported earnings (Table 68). The association between high earnings in medical school and internships in minor teaching or nonteaching hospitals—was more pronounced for 1954 than for 1950 graduates. The difference for 1954 was significant for the private school graduates (CR 3.2) and borderline for the

TABLE 67. Percentage distribution of doctors by yearly earnings in medical school, type of internship, type of school, and year of graduation

| Yearly earnings | 1950 | | | 1954 | | |
|---|---|---|---|---|---|---|
| | Rotating | Other | No response | Rotating | Other | No response |
| | | | Public | | | |
| 0-$499 | 80 | 17 | 3 (102) | 88 | 11 | 1 (133) |
| $500-$1499 | 91 | 6 | 3 (113) | 89 | 43 | 3 (192) |
| $1500- | 88 | 7 | 4 (113) | 92 | 7 | 1 (167) |
| | | | Private | | | |
| 0-$499 | 54 | 44 | 2 (205) | 49 | 50 | 1 (212) |
| $500-$1499 | 55 | 43 | 3 (112) | 54 | 45 | 1 (184) |
| $1500- | 55 | 42 | 3 (106) | 62 | 36 | 2 (111) |

TABLE 68. Percentage distribution of doctors by yearly earnings in medical school by hospital of internship, type of school, and year of graduation

| Yearly earnings | 1950 | | | | 1954 | | | |
|---|---|---|---|---|---|---|---|---|
| | Public | | Private | | Public | | Private | |
| | Major teaching | Other | Major teaching | Other | Major teaching | Other | Major teaching | Other |
| 0-$499 | 36 | 27 | 48 | 48 | 35 | 21 | 46 | 32 |
| $500-$1,499 | 32 | 35 | 25 | 28 | 37 | 39 | 36 | 35 |
| $1,500- | 30 | 37 | 25 | 23 | 26 | 39 | 17 | 32 |
| No response | 2 | 2 | 2 | 1 | 2 | 1 | 1 | 0 |
| | (132) | (199) | (278) | (149) | (210) | (285) | (354) | (154) |

public school group (CR 1.98). The absence of a similar difference for the 1950 graduates may be due to the G.I. Bill which was a frequent source of support reported by the members of that cohort.

Similarly, lower earnings are associated with the choice of a major teaching hospital for residency except among the 1950 private school graduates (Table 69). Although this tendency is quite consistent, the associations are not strong.

The frequency of reported no residency appears from Table 69 to be consistently associated with earnings during medical school. Among the differences between residency and no residency that were significant are those for 1950 public school graduates with earnings of $499 or less (CR 2.2), the 1950 private school graduates in the same income category (CR 1.9), and the 1950 public school graduates with the highest earnings (CR 2.4). None of the differences for the 1954 graduates were significant. The fact that none of the differences found for the private school groups were definitely significant may again be due to the small size of the group without residency training—37, or 8 percent of the total, in 1950 and 21, or 5 percent of the total group, in 1954.

Among doctors with a residency, the length of residency training was also associated with the history of earnings in medical school given by public school graduates (Table 70). Testing of the tendency of public school graduates with high earnings to take shorter residencies was significant for the 1950 graduates (CR 2.7) but not for those of 1954. While this tendency was also present among the private school graduates, it was neither very strong nor regular and was not significant.

The results of this closer examination of the influence of finances on training are consistent with those presented in the

TABLE 69. Percentage distribution of doctors by yearly earnings while in medical school by hospital of residency, type of school, and year of graduation

| Yearly earnings | 1950 | | | | 1954 | | | |
|---|---|---|---|---|---|---|---|---|
| | Public | | Private | | Public | | Private | |
| | Major teaching | Other | Major teaching | Other | Major teaching | Other | Major teaching | Other |
| 0-$499 | 43 | 31 | 48 | 50 | 31 | 28 | 46 | 38 |
| $500-$1,499 | 33 | 37 | 24 | 25 | 40 | 35 | 35 | 37 |
| $1,500- | 25 | 29 | 25 | 23 | 28 | 35 | 18 | 24 |
| No response | 0 | 3 | 2 | 1 | 1 | 2 | 0 | 0 |
| | (80) | (154) | (170) | (222) | (159) | (215) | (234) | (255) |

TABLE 70. Percentage distribution of doctors by yearly earnings while in medical school by months of residency and by type of school and year of graduation

| Yearly earnings | Months of residency | | | | | | |
|---|---|---|---|---|---|---|---|
| | 1950 | | | | 1954 | | |
| | None | 1-23 | 24-47 | 48- | None | 1-23 | 24-47 | 48- |
| | Public | | | | | | | |
| 0-$499 | 20 | 24 | 35 | 40 | 19 | 26 | 31 | 26 |
| $500-$1,499 | 30 | 38 | 34 | 38 | 42 | 34 | 35 | 46 |
| $1,500- | 48 | 38 | 30 | 19 | 39 | 40 | 32 | 26 |
| No response | 2 | 0 | 1 | 3 | 0 | 0 | 2 | 1 |
| | (100) | (29) | (142) | (63) | (123) | (53) | (239) | (83) |
| | Private | | | | | | | |
| 0-$499 | 30 | 46 | 50 | 50 | 33 | 35 | 43 | 41 |
| $500-$1,499 | 41 | 19 | 26 | 23 | 38 | 30 | 34 | 40 |
| $1,500- | 30 | 35 | 21 | 26 | 29 | 35 | 21 | 19 |
| No response | 0 | 0 | 2 | 1 | 0 | 0 | 1 | 0 |
| | (37) | (43) | (239) | (111) | (21) | (43) | (278) | (167) |

previous chapter. Medical students who support themselves in small or large part in medical school do not appear to differ in their intellectual accomplishments from other students, but their internships and residency are affected. Although the effects upon training may not be strong, their consistently is remarkable.

*Debt at Graduation*

We have seen that the amount of debt incurred by the time of graduation as reported by the doctors showed some variation between 1950 and 1954 and between public and private schools (Table 23). The amount reported increased in both types of schools from 1950 to 1954, a possible effect of the diminished frequency of the G.I. Bill payments in 1954 and of increases in tuition and costs of living. The proportion with minimal debt, defined as $100 or less, was slightly smaller in public than in private schools.

When debt and MCAT scores are examined, a slight tendency was noted for doctors with high scores to be drawn disproportionately from the low-debt group and vice versa. There was no consistent association between debt and class rank.

Debts incurred in obtaining a medical education might be expected to show a deterrent influence on the amount and type of training obtained in preparation for practice.

Debt at graduation appeared to be associated with the choice of a type of internship as is illustrated in Table 71. Rotating internships were associated with more frequent large debt (over $3000) and less frequent small (less than $100) or no debt. The 1954 private school graduates were the only group for whom this association was weak, and, as it proved, not significant. The differences in frequency of low debt between men with rotating

TABLE 71. Percentage distribution of doctors with rotating and straight medical or surgical internships by amount of debt at graduation, by type of school and year of graduation

| Amount of debt | Public | | | | | | | | Private | | | | | | | |
|---|---|---|---|---|---|---|---|---|---|---|---|---|---|---|---|---|
| | 1950 | | | | 1954 | | | | 1950 | | | | 1954 | | | |
| | Rotating | | Straight | | Rotating | | Straight | | Rotating | | Straight | | Rotating | | Straight | |
| 0-$100 | 64 | | 76 | | 57 | | 80 | | 66 | | 79 | | 60 | | 66 | |
| $101-$3,000 | 24 | | 24 | | 26 | | 14 | | 17 | | 9 | | 22 | | 22 | |
| $3,001- | 12 | | 0 | | 17 | | 6 | | 17 | | 12 | | 18 | | 12 | |
| | (288) | | (21) | | (439) | | (28) | | (229) | | (140) | | (267) | | (184) | |

and those with straight internships was significant for the private 1950 graduates (CR 2.3) and the public 1954 graduates (CR 2.3) and was borderline for the public 1950 group (CR 1.9). There were no real differences among the groups with intermediate-sized debts, but among those with the largest debts they were very definite. The differences in frequency of large debt between doctors with rotating and those with straight internships were significant in three of the four groups (private, 1950, CR 2.3; public, 1950, CR 7.4; and public, 1954, CR 4.1). "Other" types of internship, including mixed internships and other straight services, showed a variable relationship to debt, as the mixed character of this small group would lead one to expect.

Debt at graduation had some association with the hospital of internship (Table 72). Doctors who interned in major teaching hospitals, in most groups, were more frequently essentially debt-free at graduation than doctors who interned in other hospitals. These differences were all significant except those for the 1954 private school graduates; among the other three groups the critical ratio values ranged from 2.2 to 2.7. There was no great difference between the two internship groups in relation to large debts, and none of the small differences were significant.

The decision as to whether to obtain a residency was not constantly associated with debt at graduation (Table 73). In some groups small debts (less than $100) were more frequently associated with residency and higher debts (greater than $3000) with more frequent reporting of no residency, but this was not consistent, and in the case of the 1950 private school graduates the reverse is the case. The only significant pattern of association was that for the 1954 public school graduates, who reported no residency and also reported significantly less small debt (CR 3.3) and more large debt (CR 4.2) than doctors who reported

TABLE 72. Percentage distribution of doctors by debt at graduation and hospital of internship, by type of school and year of graduation

| Amount of debt | Public | | | | | | Private | | | |
|---|---|---|---|---|---|---|---|---|---|---|
| | 1950 | | 1954 | | 1950 | | 1954 | | | |
| | Major teaching | Other | Major teaching | Other | Major teaching | Other | Major teaching | Other | | |
| 0-$100 | 74 | 59 | 67 | 52 | 72 | 63 | 66 | 55 | | |
| $101-$3,000 | 15 | 29 | 16 | 30 | 14 | 17 | 21 | 24 | | |
| $3,001- | 10 | 12 | 16 | 16 | 12 | 19 | 13 | 19 | | |
| | (132) | (199) | (210) | (285) | (278) | (149) | (354) | (154) | | |

TABLE 73. Percentage distribution of doctors by residency or no residency and amount of debt at graduation, by type of school and year of graduation

| Amount of debt | 1950 | | | | 1954 | | | |
| --- | --- | --- | --- | --- | --- | --- | --- | --- |
| | Public | | Private | | Public | | Private | |
| | Residency | No residency | Residency | No residency | Residency | No residency | Residency | No residency |
| -$100 | 70 | 55 | 70 | 78 | 63 | 46 | 63 | 57 |
| $101-$3000 | 19 | 34 | 15 | 11 | 24 | 27 | 23 | 10 |
| $3001- | 11 | 11 | 15 | 11 | 13 | 26 | 14 | 33 |
| | (232) | (100) | (385) | (37) | (368) | (121) | (482) | (21) |

residency training. Debt thus does not seem to be a consistently important consideration in making decisions about residency training.

Debt at graduation seems to have little association with the hospital of residency. Doctors who graduated with insignificant or no debt usually obtained major teaching residencies with greater frequency than those with a larger debt. The association was not strong, however, and was absent in the case of the 1954 private school graduates. Length of residency did not appear to be associated with amount of debt at graduation.

*Medical Student Dissatisfactions*

Medical education is unusually expensive and demanding. Presumably different students will react differently to its demands; it is possible that it is not the actual demands which a student faces, but his reaction to them, that influences his preparations for practice. As we have seen, students were therefore asked whether their economic situation placed them at a disadvantage to other students in pursuit of leisure activities and purchase of clothing, food, or housing. About a third of the students felt strongly that their leisure activities were curtailed by finances, and about a quarter felt similarly about clothing. Somewhat over 10 percent were dissatisfied with their housing and about half as many felt deprivations with respect to food. When these opinions are compared with the training doctors obtained, there is little evidence that they were associated with the doctor's choice of hospital or that they affected the duration of his residency.

Doctors who were married while in medical school were asked whether their spouses had felt strongly about lack of food, housing, leisure, and clothing. The answers did not give any clear evidence that a spouse's feelings of deprivation affected the doctor's training.

Doctors were also asked whether their medical education curtailed certain social, recreational, cultural, and family activities. While many doctors and their spouses did feel that these had been curtailed, the fact seemed to have little association with their choice of subsequent training.

*Marriage*

Students who were married before entering medical school were probably older than those who were not, and more likely to have children during medical training than those who married later. Any associations that marriage may have with training or performance in school may be complicated by these other circumstances associated with marriage. Further evidence indicating selection of different students in public and private schools is furnished by the proportion who were married at the time of entering medical school. The percents for public school students were 38 and 21 in 1950 and 1954. The percents married before entering private medical schools were 26 and 13. The higher proportion of older students was in all probability the reason for the higher proportion of married students among the 1950 graduates.

Other studies of the academic records of married and single undergraduate students have found slight but nonsignificant grade differences.(14, 20, 25) In this study there was no suggestion that marriage before medical school was associated in any systematic fashion with class rank. The distribution of the public and private medical school graduates by MCAT scores was essentially similar for the married and single student. Thus, it is again found that personal or family characteristics of doctors which may influence their preparation for practice are not systematically associated with their ability or performance as judged by these conventional academic measures.

Selection of a rotating, in preference to a straight, internship was not apparently related to marriage prior to medical school. The choice of hospital of internship, however, was consistently related to early marriage, in that interns in major teaching hospitals were more often single when in medical school (Table 74). A higher proportion of doctors with "other" internships was married. Although this difference appears to be common to all groups, it proved to be significant only for the 1950 public school graduates (CR 2.4). The married private and public school graduates were not significantly different with respect to frequency of major teaching hospital internships in either 1950 or 1954—marriage prior to medical school apparently had a similar constraining influence on the decisions of both groups. The unmarried public and private school graduates, on the other hand, did report significantly different frequencies of major teaching hospital internships (CR 2.4 for 1950 and 2.3 for 1954).

A similar but weaker tendency is found when marriage and choice of the hospital of residency are examined. This trend was present in all groups but it was not strong enough to merit testing.

Residency training showed other effects related to marriage prior to medical school entrance (Table 75). The proportion of this early-married group with no residency was two to three times greater than that of the single group. These differences in frequency of no residency are significant for the private school graduates.

TABLE 74. Percentage distribution of doctors by hospital of internship and marriage before entering medical school, by type of school and year of graduation

|  | Public | | | | Private | | | |
|  | 1950 | | 1954 | | 1950 | | 1954 | |
|  | Major teaching | Other | Major teaching | Other | Major teaching | Other | Major teaching | Other |
|---|---|---|---|---|---|---|---|---|
| Married | 27 | 45 | 17 | 24 | 21 | 36 | 10 | 20 |
| Single | 73 | 54 | 82 | 76 | 78 | 64 | 90 | 80 |
|  | (132) | (199) | (210) | (285) | (278) | (149) | (354) | (154) |

TABLE 75. Percentage distribution of doctors by marriage before medical school, by months of residency, type of school, and year of graduation

| Months residency | Public | | | | Private | | | |
| --- | --- | --- | --- | --- | --- | --- | --- | --- |
| | 1950 | | 1954 | | 1950 | | 1954 | |
| | Married | Not married | Married | Not married | Married | Not married | Married | Not married |
| None | 48 | 19 | 44 | 20 | 14 | 7 | 10 | 3 |
| -23 | 9 | 8 | 11 | 10 | 12 | 9 | 12 | 8 |
| 24-47 | 28 | 52 | 35 | 51 | 55 | 56 | 49 | 55 |
| 48- | 15 | 21 | 10 | 18 | 19 | 28 | 28 | 33 |
| | (127) | (205) | (105) | (391) | (112) | (317) | (67) | (442) |

The length of residency was also associated with time of marriage. Short residencies (one to twenty-three months) were reported more often by the doctors married before medical school and than by those who were not. The groups who were married before entering medical school reported far fewer long residencies, defined here as twenty-four months or more; this difference was significant for the 1954 private school (CR 2.6), and for the public school groups (CR 5.2 for 1950 and 4.2 for 1954).

When marriage while in medical school was examined, there was no consistent difference between public and private schools. Twenty-four and 25 percent of the public and private school graduates of 1950 married while in school. These percents rose to 42 and 32 for the public and private school graduates who finished in 1954.

Marriage while a medical student showed no association with the MCAT score, nor was class rank clearly or consistently different for students who married and those who did not.

The choice of internship, which has been found to vary with most other personal characteristics, does not appear to be notably associated with marriage while in medical school. The rotating internship was reported with equal frequency by students who married and by students who remained single during medical school. Nor was hospital of internship—major teaching or other—consistently related to student marriage. The frequency of residency among the doctors who married or remained single while in medical school was not consistently different. Their distribution between major teaching and other types of residencies and in relation to length of residency was also unrelated to marriage patterns.

The consistent absence of any association of marriage while in medical school with training is striking, both because it is one of the few important personal characteristics reported by doctors that had no such association and because it contrasts so sharply with marriage contracted before entering medical school. The latter, as we have seen, is strongly associated with choice of nonteaching hospital internship, no residency, and shorter residency training. This association may be related more to age than to early marriage, but the possibility that very early marriage selects certain types of people who are impatient to enter practice (or other similar explanations) cannot be ruled out. The probability of children almost certainly increases as marriage is prolonged; this may be another constraint on longer training. The doctors who marry while in medical school apparently do not let this action influence their decisions or plans about preparation for practice. They have been at risk for a shorter period, of course, and probably have smaller families.

*The Views of Wives*

It was anticipated that married medical students would be influenced by their wives in making decisions about training, so a few questions were asked about the spouse. The first sought information on whether the spouse had been employed and a second asked whether the spouse had felt deprivation during the years of medical training with respect to food, housing, clothing, or leisure time. It must be remembered that these responses were reported by the doctors, not the wives themselves.

Seventy-four percent of the spouses of married 1950 graduates had been employed. Among 1954 graduates who were married as medical students 83 percent of the wives of public school and 87 percent of the wives of private school graduates were employed. The fact that the spouse was employed did not seem to have any definite association with the doctor's medical school performance or with his choice of training.

When doctors reported that their wives had felt strongly about their lot, it was evident their reactions varied. Less than 10 percent stated that food was a problem and about a quarter were greatly dissatisfied with their housing. A few more felt strongly about clothing. About a third of the spouses felt that leisure was curtailed. There were some suggestions that wives' attitudes may have had an effect upon the doctor's training, but these were neither large nor consistent. They bore no distinguishable relationship to the doctor's academic performance.

The decision to marry or not marry was not influenced by students' plans for their futures. Most doctors indicated that they remained single because they had not found the right person. There was no apparent relationship (among married students) between postponement of children and length of training.

*Class Esteem*

As mentioned in Chapter IV, two questions were asked to ascertain possible influence of students on one another in selecting practices and preparing for them. The first asked each doctor to indicate who his best friends were, and the second asked what classmates he would turn to for academic assistance. The data on the 1954 classes are illustrative of the responses.

Respondents were requested to give three ranked choices of fellow students they would consult about academic matters. An esteem or respect gradient has been based upon the number of first, second, and third choices received by each individual. These are arranged in classes from I, the class most respected for their ability, to IV, a class unlikely to be consulted by their fellow students. The numbers in each category are quite unequal as is evident from Table 76, which shows ratings by students of their fellows in relation to MCAT scores. Class esteem appears to be a suitable term to describe these ratings and will be used hereafter.

TABLE 76. Percentage distribution of doctors by MCAT score and class esteem ranking, by type of school, 1954 only

| MCAT score | Class esteem ranking | | | | | | | |
|---|---|---|---|---|---|---|---|---|
| | Public | | | | Private | | | |
| | I | II | III | IV | I | II | III | IV |
| 600- | 32 | 24 | 18 | 18 | 75 | 40 | 43 | 38 |
| 501-600 | 58 | 49 | 55 | 51 | 17 | 48 | 42 | 43 |
| -500 | 11 | 27 | 28 | 30 | 8 | 12 | 16 | 19 |
| | (19) | (45) | (174) | (214) | (24) | (50) | (166) | (245) |

The respect which students received from their classmates was strongly correlated with the MCAT score. It was even more closely correlated with medical school rank (Table 77). Esteem and class rank may not be independent variables; a student may be respected because his academic accomplishments are known to other students. It is, unlikely, however, that they know one another's composite MCAT scores. It is evident that students are able to make remarkably realistic judgments about one another.

The most respected individuals comprise a small and highly selected group (about 7 percent in each class), and this should be borne in mind in the following comparisons.

A larger proportion of leaders in class esteem took straight internships than their classmates (Table 78). These leaders also

TABLE 77. Percentage distribution of doctors by class rank, type of school, and class esteem ranking, 1954 only

| Class rank | Class esteem ranking | | | | | | | |
|---|---|---|---|---|---|---|---|---|
| | Public | | | | Private | | | |
| | I | II | III | IV | I | II | III | IV |
| Upper | 95 | 54 | 35 | 18 | 88 | 72 | 38 | 19 |
| Middle | 5 | 35 | 42 | 40 | 12 | 17 | 40 | 34 |
| Lower | 0 | 12 | 23 | 41 | 0 | 11 | 22 | 47 |
| | (20) | (52) | (181) | (245) | (24) | (53) | (177) | (255) |

more frequently chose major teaching hospitals for their internships and residencies than their classmates (Table 79). Furthermore, fewer esteem leaders reported no residency than their colleagues (Table 80). The length of the residencies taken by the leaders, however, was not particularly different from that taken by the other classmen.

On the basis of the named friends and the rank order of friendships in each class it was possible to identify circles of friends. Using these frequencies and rank orders it was possible

TABLE 78. Percentage distribution of class esteem leaders and other students by type of internship and type of school, 1954 only

| Type of internship | Public | | Private | |
|---|---|---|---|---|
| | Leaders | Others | Leaders | Others |
| Rotating | 82 | 90 | 27 | 55 |
| Straight and other | 18 | 8 | 73 | 43 |
| No response | 0 | 2 | 0 | 2 |
| | (33) | (465) | (37) | (472) |

TABLE 79. Percent of doctors by class esteem ranking with major teaching hospital training, 1954 only

| | Class esteem group | | | | | | | |
|---|---|---|---|---|---|---|---|---|
| | Internship | | | | Residency | | | |
| School | I | II | III | IV | I | II | III | IV |
| Public | 70 | 46 | 44 | 38 | 76 | 43 | 48 | 34 |
| | (20) | (51) | (180) | (243) | (17) | (40) | (143) | (174) |
| Private | 100 | 72 | 72 | 65 | 83 | 56 | 54 | 38 |
| | (24) | (53) | (177) | (254) | (24) | (52) | (170) | (243) |

to describe leaders and central and peripheral members within each friendship circle. In addition there were other doctors who were classed as nongroup members. These men had friends and were claimed as friend by others, but they were not clearly members of a single circle. Lastly, there were certain doctors who were apparently isolates because they claimed very few friends and were infrequently claimed as friends by other doctors and were not claimed as close friends.

The relationship of friendship groups to academic performance and hospital training yielded some interesting results.

TABLE 80. Percent of doctors by class esteem ranking with no residency, 1954 only

| School | I | II | III | IV |
|---|---|---|---|---|
| Public | 15 | 23 | 20 | 29 |
| | (20) | (52) | (181) | (245) |
| Private | 0 | 4 | 4 | 5 |
| | (24) | (53) | (177) | (225) |

Group leaders, for example, ranked higher in class standing than their followers. Similarly, a slightly higher proportion of leaders interned in major teaching hospitals than other members of a circle (Table 81). Their residency training showed the same characteristic. The followers who were central members of the group did not differ from those who were peripheral. The non-group students were different and variable with respect to the above characteristics. The isolates among the private school graduates received less and poorer training than their classmates.

TABLE 81. Percentage distribution of doctors by friendship group, by hospital of internship and type of school, 1954 only

| Hospital | Group leader | Central member | Peripheral member | Non-group | Isolated |
|---|---|---|---|---|---|
| | | | Public | | |
| Major teaching | 48 | 40 | 41 | 50 | 45 |
| Other | 52 | 60 | 59 | 50 | 55 |
| | (77) | (219) | (141) | (38) | (20) |
| | | | Private | | |
| Major teaching | 75 | 70 | 70 | 61 | 40 |
| Other | 25 | 30 | 30 | 39 | 60 |
| | (84) | (230) | (151) | (28) | (15) |

From even this brief discussion it is evident that friendships and esteem relationships have some associations with performance in medical school and with the amount and kind of hospital training a doctor receives.

## Timing of Decisions About Training

The stage of a doctor's career at which he makes his decision about how much training to obtain could be of practical importance. If, as was assumed in planning this study, more training will result in greater clinical skill, it is possible that information on the timing of decisions about training may indicate points of intervention at which less wise decisions could be altered. For example, 50 percent or more of the doctors who reported no residency made the decision about amount of training during their internship. The late date of this decision suggests that it could be changed. Since various types of internships are associated with the probability of further training, the interns most likely to terminate their training at that stage are easily identified.

The timing of the decision about total amount of training to be obtained had some relationships that would be expected. While doctors with rotating internships usually made this decision during their internship, those with straight internships most frequently made this decision while in medical school. Doctors who reported that their decisions about training were made during medical school reported straight and "other" (not rotating) internships with significantly greater frequency than doctors who reported rotating internships; the critical ratio values for these differences among public school graduates of 1950 and 1954 were 4.4 and 5.5, and those for the private school groups were 2.5 for 1950 and 4.8 for 1954. Those doctors who stated that their training decisions were made during the internship more frequently reported rotating internships. The different frequency of rotating and other internships was significant for each group (CR: public, 1950, 2.3; public, 1954, 2.2; private, 1950, 7.1; and private, 1954, 3.0).

Doctors who made their decisions about training during medical school reported a higher frequency of major teaching hospital internships than did doctors who made their decisions at other stages of their career. This difference was significant for all groups except the 1954 public school graduates, who did not differ in this distribution. The critical ratios for the other three groups ranged from 2.5 to 3.7. Doctors whose residency was in a major teaching hospital tended to report an earlier decision about total training than those with residency in other hospitals. The frequency of major teaching hospital residency was significantly greater than "other" residency for both public (CR 2.6) and private school graduates (CR 2.8) of 1950 who made their decision during medical school. Though similar differences were found in 1954, these were not so marked and they were not significant. Doctors who finally decided their training programs during their internship more often reported residencies in other than major teaching hospitals, but this reached significance only for the 1950 private school graduates (CR 2.0). Doctors who reported residencies did not show a consistent pattern of timing their training decision in relation to the length of residency.

Among all doctors about 10 percent stated that their decision was made while in medical school. About two thirds reported that it was made during medical school or internship, and the remainder made it during their residency.

*Advice and Counsel Received by Trainees*

Doctors were asked whether they had been encouraged by family members, faculty, or other individuals to continue training beyond the internship. We have seen that in general, private school graduates reported receiving encouragement more often than did public school graduates. Parents, medical school deans, student advisers, and personal physicians were the least frequent sources of encouragement. Members of clinical faculties were a more frequent source.

Doctors who had rotating internships reported that they received encouragement to continue training less frequently than did those with straight internships in all groups (Table 82).

When the various differences between doctors with rotating and straight internships were tested for significance, several different results emerged. Although the doctors who had straight internships consistently reported more encouragement from their medical and clinical teachers, the differences in the amount of encouragement which they reported and that reported by doctors with rotating internships was only occasionally significant. For example, the public school graduates of both 1950 and 1954 who had straight internships reported significantly more encouragement than graduates with rotating internships from their medical school deans and advisers (CR 6.2 and 2.8); the differences reported by the private school graduates were not significant.

In contrast, the differences between doctors with rotating and straight internships who reported parental encouragement was significant in most instances, with far more encouragement reported by those who had had straight internships. The difference was not significant for the private school 1950 graduates, but for the other groups the critical ratios ranged from 3.2 to 4. The public and private school graduates who had straight internships were not significantly different with regard to parental support in either 1950 or 1954, but the public school graduates with rotating internships received less parental support than their private school counterparts with significance values far beyond chance. The critical ratios for the 1950 public–private school difference was 6.3; for 1954 it was 4.9. Backing from a spouse

TABLE 82. Percent of doctors who were encouraged to obtain residency training by source of encouragement, by type of internship, type of school, and year of graduation

| Source of encouragement | Public | | | | Private | | | |
|---|---|---|---|---|---|---|---|---|
| | 1950 | | 1954 | | 1950 | | 1954 | |
| | Rotating | Straight | Rotating | Straight | Rotating | Straight | Rotating | Straight |
| Parents | 21 | 48 | 24 | 51 | 36 | 42 | 39 | 53 |
| Dean or adviser | 15 | 43 | 16 | 47 | 26 | 31 | 36 | 46 |
| Medical school teachers | 38 | 48 | 44 | 73 | 46 | 65 | 55 | 70 |
| Spouse | 31 | 62 | 36 | 43 | 46 | 48 | 41 | 54 |
| Attending physician | 41 | 38 | 47 | 68 | 63 | 70 | 61 | 66 |
| Clinical chief | 47 | 57 | 54 | 65 | 61 | 70 | 65 | 72 |
| Residents | 34 | 52 | 45 | 68 | 58 | 64 | 61 | 67 |
| | (290) | (21) | (446) | (37) | (234) | (142) | (271) | (184) |

was associated with choice of a rotating or straight internship in a manner very similar to that shown for parental encouragement. The 1950 private school graduates were exceptional in that there was no difference in frequency of reported encouragement between graduates with rotating and straight internships. In the other three groups of graduates the differences were substantial and significant (CR range from 3.2 to 10). Doctors with straight internships who graduated from public and private schools were not significantly different in either 1950 or 1954, whereas those who reported rotating internships were; the critical ratio was 5.3 for the 1950 and 2.5 for the 1954 difference between public and private schools in reported frequency of encouragement by a spouse.

Although the private school graduates seem to obtain substantially more encouragement from their faculty, this greater backing was irregularly associated with the choice of type of internship. The similarity of doctors in public and private schools who report straight internships and the dissimilarities between those reporting rotating internships again emphasizes the differences in students in the two types of institutions.

Doctors with the more desirable teaching-hospital training consistently reported more encouragement than those with other internships. Medical school teachers seemed to be especially selective in advising students (Table 83).

Parental encouragement was associated more frequently with major teaching hospital internships for most groups. Parental encouragement was reported significantly more often by the public (CR 3.5) and private (CR 2.9) school graduates of 1950 with major teaching hospital internships. The difference in frequency of reported encouragement by medical school teachers may bear a cause and effect relationship to the frequency of

TABLE 83. Percent of doctors who were encouraged to obtain residency training by source of encouragement, by hospital of internship, type of school and year of graduation

| Source of encouragement | Public | | | | Private | | | |
|---|---|---|---|---|---|---|---|---|
| | 1950 | | 1954 | | 1950 | | 1954 | |
| | Major teaching | Other | Major teaching | Other | Major teaching | Other | Major teaching | Other |
| Parents | 31 | 19 | 31 | 22 | 43 | 30 | 48 | 40 |
| Dean or adviser | 23 | 13 | 27 | 12 | 34 | 19 | 46 | 27 |
| Medical school teachers | 50 | 31 | 61 | 36 | 64 | 38 | 71 | 42 |
| Spouse | 36 | 32 | 38 | 35 | 50 | 42 | 48 | 44 |
| Attending physician | 41 | 40 | 51 | 47 | 67 | 61 | 63 | 60 |
| Clinical chief | 49 | 48 | 60 | 52 | 70 | 56 | 70 | 63 |
| Residents | 43 | 32 | 54 | 40 | 67 | 51 | 67 | 54 |
| | (132) | (199) | (210) | (285) | (278) | (149) | (354) | (154) |

teaching appointments. The critical ratios range from 2.8 to 4.4 for the differences in frequency of encouragement reported.

Between doctors with residency in major teaching hospitals and those in other hospitals there were some differences in frequency of encouragement in pursuing a residency. As is to be expected in this selected group, the differences are diminished as compared with those found for internship choices (Table 84).

Longer residency was associated with higher rates of reported encouragement from parents (Table 85). Calculation of the regression indicates that this association was significant for the public school graduates of both 1950 (CR 3.7) and 1954 (CR 2.1) and also for the private school graduates (CR 2.4 for 1950 and 4.5 for 1954). Encouragement from a spouse was rather regularly associated with longer residency training but this association was strong and significant (CR 7.2) only for the public school graduates of 1950.

When the advice given to students and trainees is compared with class rank, it is clear that the higher ranked students reported more encouragement from all sources than did those of lower rank (Table 86). This is true whatever the source of advice. That there is a suggestive association between the encouragement given to students by faculties and the class rank which is determined by (or, at least, known to) the same faculty is not an accidental finding. The curious thing is that the faculties neglect students (at least the students report less advice and encouragement) in lower class ranks. These students may be the ones most in need of encouragement.

When these trends are tested, only occasional significant associations are found. Parental encouragement was significantly associated with class rank for graduates of 1950, but not for graduates of 1954. Encouragement by a spouse was associated with class rank for the public school 1950 graduates (CR 4.0) but

TABLE 84. Percent of doctors who were encouraged to obtain residency training by source of encouragement and hospital of residency, by type of school and year of graduation

| Source of encouragement | Public | | | | Private | | | |
|---|---|---|---|---|---|---|---|---|
| | 1950 | | 1954 | | 1950 | | 1954 | |
| | Major teaching | Other | Major teaching | Other | Major teaching | Other | Major teaching | Other |
| Parents | 39 | 28 | 36 | 28 | 45 | 38 | 47 | 46 |
| Dean or adviser | 25 | 17 | 25 | 17 | 25 | 31 | 46 | 35 |
| Medical school teachers | 55 | 36 | 54 | 48 | 64 | 50 | 70 | 56 |
| | (80) | (154) | (159) | (215) | (170) | (222) | (234) | (255) |

TABLE 85. Percent of doctors who were encouraged to obtain residency by source of encouragement, by months of residency, type of school, and year of graduation

| Source of encouragement | Months of residency | | | | | | | |
|---|---|---|---|---|---|---|---|---|
| | 1950 | | | | 1954 | | | |
| | None | <23 | 24-47 | 48> | None | <23 | 24-47 | 48> |
| Public | | | | | | | | |
| Parents | 6 | 17 | 30 | 43 | 10 | 34 | 27 | 42 |
| Spouse | 11 | 14 | 47 | 49 | 11 | 38 | 44 | 49 |
| | (100) | (29) | (142) | (63) | (123) | (53) | (239) | (83) |
| Private | | | | | | | | |
| Parents | 11 | 28 | 41 | 45 | 10 | 37 | 41 | 59 |
| Spouse | 14 | 47 | 50 | 53 | 5 | 47 | 47 | 52 |
| | (37) | (43) | (239) | (111) | (21) | (43) | (278) | (167) |

not for other groups. Encouragement from medical school faculty and clinical preceptors was significantly but irregularly associated with class rank. Significant associations were more frequently found for the public school graduates.

The fact that more encouragement is given the brighter students is also evident when one looks at the MCAT scores received by the respondents (Table 87). There is a tendency for high-scoring students to report more frequent encouragement than low scoring students whatever the source. In many instances the differences were not great. The tendency for medical school teachers to give more encouragement to brighter students—as defined by the MCAT—was significant in the case of the public school graduates (CR 2.3) and borderline for the private school group (CR 1.9).

TABLE 86. Percent of doctors who were encouraged to obtain residency by source of encouragement and by class rank, type of school, and year of graduation

| Source of encouragement | Public | | | | | | Private | | | | | |
|---|---|---|---|---|---|---|---|---|---|---|---|---|
| | 1950 | | | 1954 | | | 1950 | | | 1954 | | |
| | Upper | Middle | Lower | Upper | Middle | Lower | Upper | Middle | Lower | Upper | Middle | Lower |
| Parents | 32 | 24 | 16 | 31 | 22 | 26 | 44 | 39 | 32 | 48 | 45 | 43 |
| Dean or adviser | 24 | 14 | 12 | 20 | 22 | 12 | 32 | 27 | 26 | 48 | 35 | 37 |
| Medical school teachers | 49 | 38 | 28 | 50 | 51 | 39 | 62 | 56 | 45 | 70 | 61 | 55 |
| Spouse | 46 | 36 | 18 | 38 | 34 | 36 | 52 | 44 | 47 | 53 | 46 | 41 |
| Attending physician | 46 | 38 | 36 | 52 | 50 | 43 | 72 | 63 | 59 | 66 | 62 | 57 |
| Clinical chiefs | 55 | 52 | 36 | 57 | 54 | 54 | 70 | 64 | 61 | 71 | 66 | 65 |
| Residents | 42 | 35 | 31 | 67 | 62 | 60 | 72 | 58 | 53 | 52 | 44 | 43 |
| | (111) | (120) | (103) | (156) | (194) | (148) | (149) | (144) | (137) | (175) | (170) | (164) |

TABLE 87. Percent of doctors who were encouraged to obtain residency by source of encouragement, MCAT scores, and type of school, 1954 only

| Source of encouragement | Public | | | Private | | |
|---|---|---|---|---|---|---|
| | 601- | 501-600 | -500 | 601- | 501-600 | -500 |
| Parents | 31 | 24 | 23 | 48 | 48 | 33 |
| Dean or adviser | 22 | 19 | 12 | 40 | 46 | 26 |
| Medical school teachers | 53 | 50 | 35 | 67 | 64 | 43 |
| Spouse | 38 | 42 | 29 | 45 | 51 | 38 |
| Attending physician | 54 | 47 | 46 | 63 | 64 | 62 |
| Clinical chief | 62 | 56 | 47 | 69 | 70 | 62 |
| Residents | 52 | 48 | 37 | 66 | 65 | 56 |
| | (87) | (238) | (127) | (201) | (203) | (81) |

Doctors were also asked whether, if they received advice, this proved to be the most important basis for their decision. Only about one in five doctors reported that this had been the case. This proportion was slightly higher among private school graduates than among public school graduates.

## Specialty Certification

Doctors were also asked whether they were certified in a specialty or intended to seek such certification. Those who answered affirmatively differed consistently from those who did not. A higher proportion of those who were in straight internships intended to obtain certification. This same association was found with both internships and residencies in major teaching hospitals. This intention was also associated slightly with higher MCAT scores and more strongly with high class rank.

# VI / How the Graduates Viewed Their Medical Training

IN THE PRECEDING CHAPTERS, circumstances relating to career and training decisions have been considered at some length. The major question which remains is: How well satisfied were the doctors with the training they did receive? If they were dissatisfied with any aspects, which phases of training were involved and how were they unsatisfactory?

## Shortcomings in Medical Education

In an effort to ascertain the overall satisfaction of respondents with their educational experiences, the following question was asked: "Do you feel that your medical education failed in any way to provide you with the knowledge and skill which you now find you need in your practice?" Responses to this question are shown in Table 88. About half of the public school graduates felt their medical education had failed in some respect to meet their

TABLE 88. Percentage distribution of doctors by dissatisfaction with medical education, by type of school and year of graduation

|  | Public | | Private | |
|---|---|---|---|---|
|  | 1950 | 1954 | 1950 | 1954 |
| Dissatisified | 52 | 50 | 42 | 35 |
| Not dissatisfied | 48 | 50 | 58 | 65 |
|  | (334) | (498) | (430) | (509) |

needs. Although fewer of the private school graduates expressed similar sentiments, the proportion indicating dissatisfactions even in these institutions was high. The greater dissatisfaction expressed by the public school graduates when compared with the private school groups was of borderline significance for the 1950 classes (CR 1.95), and significant for 1954 (CR 5.3).

The general practitioners were more frequently critical of their medical education than the specialty groups. As Table 89 shows, the majority of general practitioners in both public and private schools indicated that their medical educations had failed them in some way or other; conversely, the majority of all other graduates indicated their education was adequate. The differences between general practitioners and all others were significant for the public school graduates (CR 3.6 for 1950 and 5.9 for 1954), and for the 1954 private school graduates (CR 2.8). The responses of the private school graduates in general practice were somewhat different from the opinions of their counterparts from the public schools. While about two thirds of the public school graduates in general practice indicated some dissatisfaction with their education, only slightly over a half of those from private schools were dissatisfied. The specialists who graduated from the two groups of schools were not very different from one another, so the differences between public and private schools are determined mainly by the proportion of doctors who entered general practice.

When one turns to a consideration of how dissatisfaction relates to academic skills and training decisions, a number of interesting associations appear. There seems to be some relationship between appraised ability and dissatisfaction. In both public and private schools those students who had the highest composite MCAT scores were most frequently critical (Table 90). Testing

TABLE 89. Percentage distribution of doctors by dissatisfaction with medical education, general practitioners and all others, by type of school and year of graduation

|  | Public | | | | Private | | | |
|---|---|---|---|---|---|---|---|---|
|  | General practice | | All others | | General practice | | All others | |
|  | 1950 | 1954 | 1950 | 1954 | 1950 | 1954 | 1950 | 1954 |
| Dissatisfied | 62 | 66 | 44 | 41 | 52 | 53 | 40 | 31 |
| Not dissatisfied | 37 | 34 | 54 | 58 | 46 | 48 | 59 | 66 |
| No response | 1 | 0 | 2 | 1 | 2 | 0 | 1 | 3 |
|  | (116) | (164) | (218) | (334) | (61) | (40) | (369) | (469) |

TABLE 90. Percentage distribution of doctors by composite MCAT scores and dissatisfaction with medical education by type of school, 1954 only

|  | Public | | | Private | | |
|---|---|---|---|---|---|---|
|  | 601- | 501-600 | -500 | 601- | 501-600 | -500 |
| Dissatisfied | 59 | 48 | 46 | 37 | 31 | 26 |
| Not dissatisfied | 41 | 51 | 54 | 60 | 67 | 74 |
|  | (87) | (238) | (127) | (201) | (203) | (81) |

of this trend showed that it was significant for the private school (CR 2.6) but not for the public school graduates. In the public schools, class rank was associated with dissatisfactions with medical education; public school graduates with poorer academic records were more often critical than those with better records. In the case of the private school graduates, there was no difference by class rank.

Less relationship was apparent between type of internship training and dissatisfaction with medical education. Graduates who chose rotating and straight internships were about equally well satisfied. The type of hospital of internship appears to be more directly related to dissatisfaction for the public school graduates than for the private school graduates. The majority of public school graduates who interned in major teaching hospitals were satisfied; conversely, the majority of those who interned in other hospitals were dissatisfied (Table 91). A majority of all private school graduates were satisfied with their medical educations; there were, nevertheless, some differences between doctors who reported major teaching and "other" internships. Public school graduates who interned in other than major teaching hospitals stated dissatisfactions significantly more often in both 1950

TABLE 91. Percentage distribution of doctors by hospital of internship and dissatisfaction with medical education, by type of school and year of graduation

|  | Public | | | | Private | | | |
|---|---|---|---|---|---|---|---|---|
|  | 1950 | | 1954 | | 1950 | | 1954 | |
|  | Major teaching | All other | Major teaching | All other | Major teaching | All other | Major teaching | All other |
| Dissatisfied | 42 | 57 | 45 | 53 | 44 | 38 | 29 | 44 |
| Not dissatisfied | 58 | 43 | 55 | 47 | 56 | 62 | 71 | 56 |
|  | (130) | (198) | (208) | (285) | (273) | (149) | (344) | (152) |

(CR 3.2) and 1954 (CR 2.5). The differences for the private school graduates were significant for 1954 (CR 3.5) but not for 1950.

Those graduates with no residency training were more often dissatisfied than those who had some residency (Table 92). The difference in frequency of dissatisfaction reported by the public school graduates with residency and those with no residency was significant in both 1950 (CR 4.5) and in 1954 (CR 4.4). The private school graduates were not significantly different. This lack of significance is related to the small numbers without residencies, thirty-seven or 9 percent in the 1950 classes and twenty-one or 4 percent among the 1954 graduates.

The frequency of dissatisfactions about medical education were found to decrease regularly with increasing length of residency—except for the 1954 graduates of private schools who did not show this negative association (Table 93). Testing this trend by regression analysis showed that there was a significant negative association between frequency of dissatisfaction and the length of residency. The critical ratio values for the different groups are: public, 1950, 2.5; public, 1954, 4.9; and private, 1950, 2.0.

From these many associations it is clear that dissatisfaction with medical education is related to and modified by hospital training.

*Reasons for Shortcomings in Medical Education*

Those respondents who said that their medical school education had failed them in some way were asked how it had failed. A wide variety of answers were received, almost all of which

TABLE 92. Percent of doctors with residency and no residency by dissatisfaction with medical education, by type of school and year of graduation

|  | Public | | | | Private | | | |
|---|---|---|---|---|---|---|---|---|
|  | 1950 | | 1954 | | 1950 | | 1954 | |
|  | Residency | No residency | Residency | No residency | Residency | No residency | Residency | No residency |
| Dissatisfied | 44 | 64 | 45 | 63 | 41 | 49 | 32 | 52 |
| Not dissatisfied | 55 | 32 | 55 | 36 | 58 | 49 | 65 | 48 |
|  | (334) | (100) | (498) | (123) | (430) | (37) | (509) | (21) |

TABLE 93. Percent of doctors dissatisfied with medical eduation, by months of residency, type of school, and year of graduation

|  | Months of residency | | |
|---|---|---|---|
|  | 1-23 | 24-47 | 48- |
| Public 1950 | 64 ( 28) | 43 (142) | 40 ( 63) |
| Public 1954 | 74 ( 53) | 43 (237) | 33 ( 83) |
| Private 1950 | 51 ( 41) | 42 (237) | 35 (111) |
| Private 1954 | 31 ( 42) | 35 (274) | 29 (160) |

could be categorized under one of the following: desired more emphasis on clinical training; desired more basic science (biochemistry, biophysics, data computing, and so forth) and more research; desired more emphasis on specialty training; desired more training in the economics and administration of medical practice; desired more psychiatric and psychosomatic training; desired more patient contact and responsibility; desired better teaching or guidance (institutional criticism); desired more emphasis on medical ethics, the art of medicine, and the relation of medicine to the humanities. The more common criticisms are listed in Table 94. This table shows the distribution of criticisms among doctors who did complain, and refers only to the principal criticism made by each complaining physician. It will be recalled that the proportions of doctors who felt that their medical education had failed in some respect were greater among the public school graduates.

The most common complaints were that the medical school failed to provide enough clinical training and—somewhat surprisingly—gave insufficient attention to the economics and ad-

TABLE 94. Percent distribution of all doctors and general practitioners by major criticism of medical education (doctors stating criticism only), by type of school and year of graduation

| Criticism | All doctors | | | | General practitioners | | | |
|---|---|---|---|---|---|---|---|---|
| | Public | | Private | | Public | | Private | |
| | 1950 | 1954 | 1950 | 1954 | 1950 | 1954 | 1950 | 1954 |
| Clinical training | 22 | 29 | 21 | 18 | 30 | 42 | 38 | 29 |
| Specialty emphasis | 16 | 22 | 10 | 9 | 16 | 18 | 9 | 10 |
| Economics and administration | 25 | 19 | 33 | 22 | 26 | 17 | 41 | 38 |
| Institutional criticism | 11 | 11 | 12 | 15 | 11 | 11 | 6 | 10 |
| Psychiatry | 9 | 9 | 11 | 19 | 8 | 5 | 3 | 14 |
| Other | 17 | 10 | 13 | 18 | 9 | 7 | 3 | 0 |
| | (174) | (254) | (181) | (176) | (76) | (112) | (32) | (21) |

ministration of medical practice. The desire for greater emphasis on specialty training is more characteristic of the public than the private schools; private school graduates almost all enter specialty practice. The private school graduates are somewhat more concerned with the adequacy of their training in psychiatry and psychosomatic medicine. With these exceptions there is remarkable uniformity of dissatisfaction among those physicians with criticisms in the public and private schools and in 1950 and 1954.

From 52 to 67 percent of general practitioners in the various groups expressed criticisms of their medical education, compared with 31 percent to 41 percent of other doctors. The differences between general practitioners and all others were significant for all groups except the 1950 private school graduates; among the other groups the critical ratio values ranged from 2.8 to 5.9. Since general practitioners were more dissatisfied with their educations than other respondents, their criticisms are included in Table 94. Here even a higher proportion of respondents felt that inadequate attention had been given to clinical training and to the economics and administration of medical practice. The private school graduates were particularly concerned about the latter. Why general practitioners graduated from public and private schools would have somewhat different feelings about specialty teaching and economics is not easily explained. The important fact is that those in general practice, who differed from their fellow doctors in a number of ways—including the brevity of their clinical training—were more often critical of their medical education.

Finally, there is the question of whether academic ability or performance bears any relation to the type of criticism expressed about medical education. In general, those respondents with the higher composite MCAT scores were the most critical. Public school graduates with high and low MCAT differed in the type of criticisms they made. Criticisms by doctors with high MCAT scores dealt chiefly with economics and administration and with general institutional shortcomings, while doctors with medium or low MCAT scores were concerned with the need for more specialty training (Table 95). Among the private school graduates, those with higher MCAT scores were more frequently critical, but there were no associations between specific criticisms and MCAT scores.

TABLE 95. Percentage distribution of doctors stating criticism by composite MCAT scores and by major criticism (public school graduates, 1954)

| Criticism | 601- | 501-600 | -500 |
|---|---|---|---|
| Clinical training | 22 | 32 | 28 |
| Specialty emphasis | 13 | 23 | 31 |
| Economics and administration | 28 | 15 | 16 |
| Institutional criticism | 19 | 9 | 7 |
| Other | 18 | 21 | 18 |
|  | (54) | (118) | (61) |

As noted previously, the grades respondents received in medical school did not have any consistent relationship to their satisfaction or dissatisfaction with medical education. But did students in the upper, middle, and lower third of the class emphasize different criticisms? In the public schools the lower ranked students were more concerned with the adequacy of the clinical training than were other students (Table 96). No other rank-related differences in criticism were found. In the private school groups academic rank was not related in any consistent manner with any of the criticisms made about medical education.

TABLE 96. Percent of doctors dissatisfied with clinical training by academic rank (public school graduates only)

|  | Upper third | Middle third | Lower third |
|---|---|---|---|
| 1950 | 5 (111) | 12 (120) | 19 (103) |
| 1954 | 5 (156) | 18 (194) | 20 (148) |

## Adequacy of Hospital Training

In addition to their evaluations of training in medical school, respondents were asked to evaluate the adequacy of their hospital training. These responses contrasted with the frequent criticisms voiced about medical education. Overall, 80 percent or more of the doctors were satisfied with their internships and residencies. There was little difference between the private and public school graduates or between those who graduated in 1950 or 1954. Eighty-six percent of the private school graduates of 1950 and 1954 expressed satisfaction with their hospital training; the corresponding percentages for the public schools were 78 and 83. When these statistics are examined by respondent's specialty, it is evident that the general practitioners (the group most dissatisfied with medical education) were also less satisfied with their hospital training than any specialty group (Table 97). The differences in frequency of dissatisfactions between general practitioners and other doctors were significant for the public school classes of 1950 (CR 3.4) and 1954 (CR 6.4), borderline for the private school 1950 classes (CR 1.9), and not significant

TABLE 97. Percent of general practitioners and all other doctors dissatisfied with hospital training, by type of school and year of graduation

|  | Public | | Private | |
|---|---|---|---|---|
|  | 1950 | 1954 | 1950 | 1954 |
| General practitioners | 34 (116) | 30 (164) | 21 (61) | 28 (40) |
| All others | 14 (218) | 10 (334) | 12 (369) | 12 (469) |

for the 1954 private school graduates. The failure of the large differences in proportions shown by this last group to reach significance is probably due to the small number (11) of general practitioners involved.

Criticisms of hospital training appeared to bear some relation to academic potential as measured by the MCAT, but none to academic performance as evidenced by grades in medical school. In the private schools the respondents with the higher MCAT scores were more critical of the adequacy of their hospital training. Although the public school graduates with the highest scores were most frequently critical, the association is otherwise not consistent or strong (Table 98). When responses to the question were ordered according to the academic rankings of the respondents in medical school, there was no tendency for those with high or low rank to be more or less satisfied with their hospital training.

Little relation was found between the internship reported and criticisms of hospital training. Doctors who interned in major teaching or other types of hospitals were about equally critical of their training. Although respondents who had obtained rotating internships were consistently more critical than those with straight internships, the differences were too slight to support any conclusions.

TABLE 98. Percentage distribution of doctors by opinion about hospital training by MCAT score (1954) and by type of school

| Training | Public | | | Private | | |
|---|---|---|---|---|---|---|
| | 601- | 501-600 | -500 | 601- | 501-600 | -500 |
| Dissatisfied | 23 | 11 | 19 | 18 | 11 | 7 |
| Satisfied | 76 | 88 | 80 | 82 | 88 | 93 |
| No response | 1 | 0 | 1 | 0 | 0 | 0 |
| | (87) | (238) | (127) | (201) | (203) | (81) |

When doctors with residency and no residency are compared, the frequency of their dissatisfactions are quite different (Table 99). These differences are significant for the public school graduates of both 1950 (CR 4.4) and 1954 (CR 6.3) and for the private school graduates of 1950 (CR 2.4) but not of 1954.

When dissatisfactions with hospital training are examined in relation to the amount of residency reported it is evident that dissatisfactions are reported more frequently by doctors whose training was short—less than twenty-four months (Table 100). Doctors with intermediate amounts of residency were not very different from those with more prolonged training (forty-eight

TABLE 99. Percent of doctors with residency or no residency who were dissatisfied with hospital training, by type of school and year of graduation

| Year | Public | | Private | |
|---|---|---|---|---|
| | Residency | No residency | Residency | No residency |
| 1950 | 14 (232) | 37 ( 99) | 12 (389) | 31 ( 36) |
| 1954 | 12 (373) | 31 (122) | 13 (487) | 33 ( 21) |

TABLE 100. Percent of doctors dissatisfied with hospital training by months of residency, type of school, and year of graduation

|  |  | Months of residency | |
|---|---|---|---|
|  | 1-23 | 24-47 | 48- |
| Public  1950 | 28 ( 29) | 12 (142) | 11 ( 63) |
| 1954 | 28 ( 53) | 10 (239) | 5 ( 83) |
| Private 1950 | 23 ( 43) | 10 (239) | 9 (111) |
| 1954 | 26 ( 43) | 11 (278) | 13 (167) |

months or more). The differences between doctors with less than two years of training and all those with longer training (twenty-four months or more) was significant for all groups except the public school 1950 graduates. The critical ratio values for the other classes were: private, 1950, 2.4; private, 1954, 2.0; and public, 1954, 4.5.

When hospital criticisms were tabulated by the type of hospital of residency, it was found that doctors who obtained their training in major teaching hospitals were neither more nor less critical than those who received their training in other hospitals.

## Reasons for Curtailing Training

From the above discussion, it is obvious that criticism of hospital training was inversely related to the amount of training received. The next question is then: What prevented the critical respondents from getting more training? Some 26 and 17 percent of the 1950 and 1954 public school graduates and 15 and 13 percent of the corresponding graduates of private schools felt that their training was curtailed; reports of the major factors responsible for this are presented in Table 101. Obviously, economic pressures constituted the most common reason for failing to obtain as much training as desired. Nearly 50 percent of the respondents were deterred by economic reasons, except in the case of the 1954 graduates of private schools. In this group about one third stated they had not yet completed their training or had plans to obtain more; changes in these plans could bring the figure for this group more closely into line with those of the graduates of 1950. It should be noted, however, that a higher proportion of these 1954 respondents were critical of the quality of their training or were anxious to get into practice than was true of the 1950 private school classes.

Since more general practitioners indicated they felt their hospital training was unsatisfactory than other respondents, it is pertinent to compare their reasons for not getting more training

TABLE 101. Percentage distribution of doctors reporting limitations of training by major responsible factor, by type of school and year of graduation

| Factor limiting | Public | | Private | |
|---|---|---|---|---|
| | 1950 | 1954 | 1950 | 1954 |
| Economic pressures | 51 | 48 | 48 | 29 |
| Military | 4 | 4 | 8 | 3 |
| Family circumstances | 13 | 8 | 12 | 14 |
| Poor quality of training | 4 | 9 | 2 | 8 |
| Tired of school, wanted to begin practice, etc. | 14 | 8 | 3 | 13 |
| Training not completed or intend more | 14 | 22 | 27 | 33 |
| | (77) | (85) | (60) | (72) |

(Table 102). From 15 to 19 percent of those in general practice who stated that they had failed to complete their desired training attributed this to economic pressures. Economic pressures were definitely less for all other doctors; they reported that economic problems were responsible for shortcomings of their training from one fifth to half as frequently as did general practitioners. These differences reached significance only for the 1954 public school graduates (CR 3.9); the difference shown by the 1950 private school graduates was borderline (CR 1.9). The public school graduates of 1950 in general practice were more frequently married before entering medical school than were doctors in any other of the three groups. Marriage before medical school, which had associations with shorter hospital training, may well have been the reason that family problems were listed more often by this group as a deterrent to training.

It should also be observed that a higher percent of general practitioners than other doctors in the private schools indicated that poor quality of training was the reason which deterred them from getting more training. Those in general practice, more than other respondents, terminated their training because they were tired of school and anxious to get into practice. Finally, a higher proportion of general practitioners than other doctors—25 to 38 percent as compared to 10 to 14 percent—acknowledged that their training had been curtailed. A substantial majority apparently did not feel that their training was abbreviated, even though, by comparison with other doctors, their residency experiences were infrequent and brief.

The relationship of hospital of residency to statements about economic pressures is fairly consistent in both public and private schools. With the exception of the private school 1954 classes, respondents who trained in other than major teaching hospitals

TABLE 102. Percentage distribution of general practitioners and all other doctors by frequency of curtailment of training, by responsible factor, by type of school, and by year of graduation

| Responsible factor | 1950 | | | | 1954 | | | |
|---|---|---|---|---|---|---|---|---|
| | Public | | Private | | Public | | Private | |
| | General practice | All other | General practice | All other | General practice | All other | General practice | All other |
| Economic pressures | 19 | 8 | 18 | 5 | 18 | 3 | 15 | 3 |
| Military | 2 | 0 | 2 | 1 | 1 | 0 | 0 | 0 |
| Family circumstances | 7 | 1 | 2 | 2 | 2 | 1 | 3 | 2 |
| Poor quality of training | 0 | 1 | 0 | 0 | 4 | 0 | 5 | 1 |
| Tired of school, wanted to begin practice, etc. | 7 | 1 | 0 | 1 | 4 | 0 | 5 | 1 |
| Training not completed or intend more | 3 | 4 | 3 | 4 | 3 | 4 | 0 | 5 |
| No comment | 63 | 84 | 75 | 88 | 68 | 90 | 73 | 87 |
| | (116) | (218) | (61) | (369) | (164) | (334) | (40) | (471) |

were more often deterred from continuing their training by economic circumstances than those in major teaching institutions. The differences in the other three groups were quite marked, but the small numbers made it impossible to accept the differences as proved.

The importance of economic pressures as a reason for curtailing training is strongly suggested when responses of public school graduates are looked at in relation to amount of residency training received. The percent of doctors who curtailed their training because of economic problems was greatest among those with the least residency. Each increment in months of residency was accompanied by a smaller percent of doctors who reported that their training was affected by economic circumstances. The small numbers involved make it impossible to give much weight to this interesting finding. A very similar result was found in the case of private school graduates who reported curtailment of training.

A quarter and a third of the doctors with less than two years of residency who received less training than planned stated that family considerations were responsible. When training was longer, family problems seldom were influential. While this association was very regular, the small numbers concerned again made any conclusions impossible.

In summary, the strongest expressed deterrent to additional training for the public school graduates was economic pressure, while for the private school graduates both economic and family circumstances were important to a small group of doctors.

*Training Choices in Retrospect*

Having considered respondents' criticisms of their hospital training, it is now appropriate to examine what kind of internship and residency training they would prefer to receive if they had the opportunity to repeat their experience. The great majority of respondents were either satisfied with their internship or made no comment to this question. Over 50 percent of the 1950 graduates and about two thirds of the 1954 graduates said they would take the same training again. The doctors who failed to comment—overall, about 20 percent—were probably not greatly dissatisfied with their experiences (Table 103). The public school graduates were somewhat better satisfied with the type of their internship but were slightly more critical of the quality of the training. A larger percent of the private school graduates, on the other hand, would have preferred a different type of internship than that received; the majority of these respondents said they would have preferred a rotating internship. Since a large majority of public school graduates did receive rotating internships, it is obvious that this type of internship was highly valued by the graduates of both public and private schools.

Surgeons who graduated from public medical schools seemed to be consistently more satisfied with their internship than other

TABLE 103. Percentage distribution of doctors choosing the same or different training by type of school and year of graduation

| Preferred internship | Public | | Private | |
|---|---|---|---|---|
| | 1950 | 1954 | 1950 | 1954 |
| Same | 56 | 67 | 55 | 63 |
| Same, but better | 8 | 10 | 6 | 5 |
| Different | 10 | 5 | 17 | 14 |
| No comment | 23 | 17 | 22 | 17 |
| Other | 2 | 1 | 1 | 1 |
| | (334) | (498) | (430) | (509) |

respondents. The private school graduates who became surgeons did not differ from their classmates (Table 104).

The graduates from the public schools who said they would have preferred the "same but better" internships represented a wide variety of specialties. It is difficult to say that one specialty was more critical than any other. The same is true for the respondents from the private schools who indicated they would have preferred a rotating internship to the one they received.

When respondents' answers as to preferred internship training are compared with the type actually received, the approval of the rotating internship is apparent (Table 105). Most of the public school graduates who preferred the same type of internship or the "same but better" reported rotating internships. A few more of the private school graduates who took straight or other internships would have preferred different training than was the case with those who took rotating internships. It should also be noted that the largest proportion of public school respondents who preferred a different internship from that actually received had had straight internship training. The numbers in these groups are, of course, very small.

Finally, when responses about preferred internship training

TABLE 104. Percent of doctors preferring the same internship as received by field of practice, by type of school and year of graduation

|  | Public | | Private | |
| --- | --- | --- | --- | --- |
|  | 1950 | 1954 | 1950 | 1954 |
| General practice | 53 (116) | 68 (164) | 49 (61) | 58 (40) |
| Medicine | 54 (52) | 61 (75) | 57 (74) | 61 (105) |
| Surgery | 66 (50) | 75 (64) | 62 (94) | 69 (122) |
| All others | 57 (116) | 65 (195) | 53 (201) | 63 (242) |

TABLE 105. Percentage distribution of doctors by type of internship received and type preferred, by type of school and year of graduation

| Preferred internship | Public | | | | | | Private | | | | | |
| --- | --- | --- | --- | --- | --- | --- | --- | --- | --- | --- | --- | --- |
| | 1950 | | 1954 | | | | 1950 | | | 1954 | | |
| | Rotating | Straight * | Rotating | Straight | * | Rotating | Straight | Other | Rotating | Straight | Other |
| Same | 58 | 48 | 68 | 57 | | 56 | 57 | 47 | 66 | 64 | 53 |
| Same, but better | 9 | 0 | 10 | 3 | | 8 | 4 | 0 | 4 | 5 | 9 |
| Different | 9 | 19 | 5 | 16 | | 13 | 17 | 31 | 12 | 15 | 19 |
| No comment | 22 | 33 | 17 | 24 | | 23 | 21 | 22 | 17 | 16 | 19 |
| Other | 0 | 0 | 0 | 0 | | 0 | 1 | 0 | 1 | 1 | 0 |
| | (290) | (21) | (446) | (37) | | (234) | (142) | (45) | (271) | (184) | (47) |

* "Other" group omitted; less than 12 responses.

are viewed in terms of the type of hospital in which respondents actually interned, the major teaching hospital is somewhat more frequently viewed as a satisfactory internship than are the other hospitals. Doctors who interned in a major teaching hospital preferred the same type of internship as that received more frequently than those who interned in another hospital in all groups except the 1954 private school graduates. The differences present in the other three groups were not great, however.

Respondents were also asked to indicate what residency training they would select if they could repeat their training experience. Responses to this question included not only those who actually received residency training but also those with none. As indicated in Table 106, 40 to 55 percent of the doctors in the several groups would have repeated their residency experience. Five to eight percent would have preferred more training and 14 to 17 percent would have selected different training.

Responses to the question varied by the specialty of the re-

TABLE 106. Percentage distribution of doctors by preferred residency, by type of school and year of graduation

| Residency preferred | Public | | Private | |
|---|---|---|---|---|
| | 1950 | 1954 | 1950 | 1954 |
| Same as received | 40 | 51 | 47 | 55 |
| Same, but better | 12 | 10 | 11 | 12 |
| Same, but more | 8 | 5 | 7 | 6 |
| Different | 17 | 15 | 15 | 14 |
| No comment | 23 | 19 | 20 | 13 |
| | (334) | (498) | (430) | (509) |

spondent. When general practitioners are compared with internists and surgeons, for example, it may be observed that a lower percent of general practitioners and higher percent of surgeons said they would repeat the training they had received than the two other specialties with which they were compared (Table 107). From Table 112 it is also apparent that it is primarily the

TABLE 107. Percentage distribution of doctors by preferred residency, by field of practice, by type of school, and by year of graduation

| Residency Preferred | 1950 | | | 1954 | | |
|---|---|---|---|---|---|---|
| | General practice | Medicine | Surgery | General practice | Medicine | Surgery |
| *Public* | | | | | | |
| Same | 22 | 40 | 58 | 29 | 52 | 69 |
| Same, but better | 5 | 13 | 14 | 5 | 9 | 14 |
| Same, but more | 9 | 10 | 2 | 11 | 3 | 2 |
| Different | 32 | 15 | 8 | 27 | 15 | 5 |
| No comment | 32 | 21 | 18 | 27 | 21 | 11 |
| | (116) | (52) | (50) | (164) | (75) | (64) |
| *Private* | | | | | | |
| Same | 38 | 49 | 57 | 38 | 49 | 64 |
| Same, but better | 5 | 16 | 15 | 5 | 10 | 15 |
| Same, but more | 13 | 3 | 3 | 10 | 9 | 2 |
| Different | 21 | 19 | 11 | 35 | 21 | 5 |
| No comment | 23 | 14 | 14 | 13 | 11 | 14 |
| | (61) | (74) | (94) | (40) | (105) | (122) |

TABLE 108. Percentage distribution of doctors by preferred residency and by months of residency, by type of school and year of graduation

| Residency preferred | Public | | | | | | Private | | | | | |
|---|---|---|---|---|---|---|---|---|---|---|---|---|
| | 1950 | | | 1954 | | | 1950 | | | 1954 | | |
| | 1-23 | 24-47 | 48- | 1-23 | 24-47 | 48- | 1-23 | 24-47 | 48- | 1-23 | 24-47 | 48- |
| Same | 24 | 49 | 57 | 40 | 64 | 63 | 47 | 51 | 51 | 49 | 57 | 58 |
| Same, but better | 7 | 17 | 16 | 13 | 11 | 11 | 9 | 12 | 13 | 9 | 13 | 11 |
| Same, but more | 31 | 7 | 3 | 19 | 2 | 5 | 7 | 8 | 4 | 10 | 5 | 8 |
| Different | 17 | 12 | 3 | 21 | 9 | 6 | 14 | 12 | 15 | 23 | 13 | 9 |
| No comment | 21 | 15 | 21 | 8 | 13 | 16 | 23 | 18 | 16 | 9 | 13 | 14 |
| | (29) | (142) | (63) | (53) | (239) | (83) | (43) | (239) | (111) | (43) | (278) | (167) |

general practitioners who would have preferred more training, and the internists and surgeons who wanted better training. Also, as would be expected, a higher percent of general practitioners than internists or surgeons would have preferred different training. Undoubtedly, some of these respondents had received no residency training and were not entirely happy about this fact.

The type of hospital in which the residency training was received showed some suggestive relationships to satisfaction with training. A larger percent of respondents who received their residencies in major teaching hospitals would select the same training than those who had taken their residencies in other hospitals. Residency in all other hospitals was more frequently associated with a desire for more and better residencies. These differences, though consistent, were not great.

As would be expected, preferred residency training is related to the amount of residency training actually received. Those who had two years or more training tend more frequently to state they would prefer the same training as they received (Table 108). Those respondents with less than two years of residency training tended more frequently to select the same but more training or different training than did respondents with two years or more of residency training. It will be noted, however, that these associations are not entirely consistent for all classes.

# VII / Discussion and Conclusion

As we stated at the onset of this volume, the present study is concerned with the differences between the doctors who prepare "well" for practice and those who do not and, more specifically, it is concerned with the characteristics of the doctor which may be associated with his decision to obtain a "good" hospital training or his decision to enter practice with minimal training. The reason for this concern is, of course, the finding in several other studies that for the great majority of physicians, longer training and training in teaching hospitals is associated with greater clinical competence. Among the questions that remained to be explored was whether this greater competence reflects the additional training—or whether the doctors who select longer training were more competent, or were different in some other significant way, to begin with. Thus, we have been concerned with such questions as: Who chooses longer training and who chooses less? Why? Who chooses teaching hospitals and who does not? Why? What are the roles of personal variables—intellectual, financial, family background, and the like—in these choices? How are all these variables related? It is now our task to examine how and to what extent we have answered these questions and to consider some of the possible implications of our findings.

The respondents in the present study came to medical school from varied backgrounds. Their fathers' educations varied from brief to long. They were drawn from all ethnic backgrounds, and more than a negligible number were born outside the United States. While most entered medical school in their early twenties, many were older. Most were single, but some were married

# DISCUSSION AND CONCLUSION

and had the additional family burden of rearing children. Their financial resources were no less varied. It was not a great surprise to find that they were disproportionately drawn from the families of physicians. Although there are less than 300,000 physicians among the nearly 200 million persons in the United States, almost 10 percent of our respondents were the sons of physicians. Neither was it surprising to learn that students from lower socioeconomic backgrounds were underrepresented. The skewed distribution of occupational background of family, of financial resources, of parents' education, and, hence, of emphasis on education and aspiration for postgraduate and professional training for a succeeding generation is apparently as true of medical education as it is of other categories of training.

These diverse variables of family backgrounds bore remarkably little relationship to the performance of students in medical school, to students' intellectual abilities as measured either by MCAT or class rank, or to other aspects of undergraduate medical education. For example, ability in medical school is not strongly associated with family background or with something as specific as the education of the student's father. Despite the diversity of backgrounds, the students who enter medical school are homogeneous with respect to intellectual ability; one may conclude that the medical schools do a very good job indeed of selecting candidates from diverse backgrounds who can make their way successfully through an undergraduate medical education.

Diversity reappears, however—and with a vengeance—when the student begins to make the critical decisions and choices regarding internships, residency, field of practice, type and length of training. These diverse patterns of decision and choice were the substrate of our investigation. Our data show that as career diversity reappears, personal and family background variables reappear as important correlates of this diversity. For example, while fathers' education had no relationship to class rank or MCAT score at medical school, it was associated with certain aspects of postgraduate medical training.

Thus, as we have seen, the students' choices of (or selection for) major teaching hospital or other hospital internships, rotating or straight internships, residency or no residency, and longer or shorter training were associated with family background, finances, academic record, MCAT score, age, marital status, and plans for practice. Indeed, even the timing of decisions about length and type of training was associated with these family, social, demographic, and personal variables.

The same family and student characteristics that were associated with choice of internship also were associated with the residency. Since doctors who had obtained a residency had undergone a second selection (and self-selection), it might be expected that these relationships would diminish, and this was found to be true. The relationship, for example, of finances or family background and the frequency of major teaching hospital residency was definitely less marked than the relationship of these variables to the type of internship. Nevertheless, several factors played an important associated role and among these, financial background seems to be of particular importance. The longer the residency training, for example, the greater the frequency of parental support of the physician in training. Of those who had four or more years of residency training, 80 percent had parental financial support for the major part of their educational costs; of those who had no residency training, only 50 percent had parental financial support of this magnitude. Conversely, the longer the residency training, the less frequently did the student report self-support.

## DISCUSSION AND CONCLUSION

What we are describing is, we believe, an interaction between a social system, a medical educational system, and a postgraduate training system. The social system produces as successful candidates for entry into medical school several distinct sets of individuals (though mainly from a fairly narrow social range)—differing in age; family, social, and educational background; financial resources; and the overall nature of their interests. These different groups of students have somewhat different careers in medical school, particularly with regard to class rank, the amount and type of encouragement they receive, and the sources of their financial support; and this experience differs somewhat in public and in private medical schools. Finally, these different sets of students make widely varying choices of internship training, and these choices tend to be the first switching points that lead on to well-defined training patterns—some longer and in prestigious teaching centers, others much shorter and in nonteaching hospitals.

Thus, one may hypothesize that clinical competence is not related to longer training alone, nor solely to self-selection for longer training by students who are different to begin with—but to both factors, interacting in a well-defined pattern.

Consider, for example, the general practitioners. Fewer of them are in the youngest age group and more of them are in the higher age group at the time of entry into medical school. Far more of them are married at the time of entry into medical school than is the case with all other doctors. They continue to marry during their medical education at the same rate as other medical students, so at the time of graduation far more of them are married. Since more are married and they have been married for a longer time, it is very probable that their family obligations are greater than those of other students. The fathers of general practitioners tend to have somewhat less education than the fathers of other doctors, and there is a tendency for these fathers to be less frequently members of the professional and executive groups that are characterized by high average incomes, and more frequently to come from families with low average income occupations. Unlike other doctors, who are born more frequently in the large and medium-sized cities of our country, general practitioners were born more frequently in small cities, towns, and rural areas.

They differ in other important respects as well. The student who is likely to become a general practitioner is overrepresented in the group with low MCAT scores and is less likely than other students to have a high MCAT score. In medical school he is more likely to rank in the lowest third of the class. He is also less likely to have been supported by his parents and more likely to have been supported by his own earnings and to have higher earnings during medical school. He reports that he received less encouragement with regard to his choice of a training program and less encouragement to continue his training from almost every source—parents, spouse, medical school, and clinical teachers.

In making his decisions about a field of practice, he is much more likely to be influenced by an interest in patients, by financial and social problems, and by his spouse, and much less likely than other doctors to report the influence of intellectual interests.

Then he is much more likely to choose a rotating internship than a straight internship; less likely to intern in a major teaching hospital and more likely to intern in a nonteaching hospital. He is more likely to have planned an internship only; but in any case, unlike other doctors, he is likeliest to make his final decision about total amount and type of training during his internship. He is far more likely than other doctors to terminate his training with internship, and obtain no residency; if he does obtain residency training, it is more likely to be in a nonteaching hospital, and to be only half as long, on the average, as the residency training obtained by other doctors. He is much more likely to cite economic and family reasons for curtailing his training.

On completion of his training, he is much more likely than other doctors to enter solo practice—indeed, he appears to represent the great stronghold of solo practice—and is less likely to be in hospital practice. He will earn a higher income sooner than his colleagues, but this income advantage will disappear within a few years.

He is substantially more likely than other doctors to be critical, in retrospect, of his undergraduate medical education (though the rate of such criticism is substantial among all doctors), particularly with regard to the quality of his undergraduate clinical training. But the general practitioner is unhappy twice over; while 80 percent of all doctors retrospectively report satisfaction with their internships and residency, the general practitioner is likely to be less satisfied with his hospital training, and to cite poor quality of training and anxiety to begin practice as reasons for curtailing it. Finally, he is more likely than physicians in other fields of practice to feel, in retrospect, that he needed more training.

This is presumably the same general practitioner who is more likely—as in the numerous studies cited earlier—to be found low in clinical competence. To associate this finding merely with length of hospital training or to presume it will be remedied merely by the prescription of more clinical training, is, in view of our data, a wildly optimistic oversimplification.

In contrast, the future medical school teacher or researcher represents another distinct set of undergraduates—and a group almost antipodal to the general practitioner. The teachers and researchers, for example, had fathers who were somewhat better educated and more frequently were professional men than were the fathers of all doctors. The doctors who went into teaching and research often were born in a large city, were younger than their classmates, and had high MCAT scores. In making their decision about a field of practice, the teachers and research workers were influenced more by intellectual interest than were any other group of doctors. Conversely, the influence of finances upon decisions about training and a field of practice was reported less frequently by these physicians than by other doctors. This group also made the decisions about their careers early, often before they came to medical school. In contrast with the general practitioners, who had many problems in obtaining a medical education, this group seemed to be a favored group. A concrete expression of this is the greater frequency with which they were recipients of scholarships. They had fewer difficulties than other doctors and many fewer problems than the general practitioners.*

* A comparison of these two polar groups—general practitioners and teachers-researchers—or of the general practitioners and the specialists does not exhaust the differences which are characteristic of physicians who selected different fields of practice. For example, the internists' academic rank was mostly skewed toward the top of their classes, they were greatly influenced by their intellectual interests, and they were seldom hampered by finances; they greatly resembled the teachers and researchers in several respects. Pediatricians' choices of a field of practice were more often influenced by interest in certain types of patients than doctors in any other type of practice, they tended to rank in the middle third of their medical school classes, and they reported shorter residencies than other specialists. Obstetrician-gynecologists, not unexpectedly, were also influenced more than other physicians by special patient interests. Surgeons reported less interest in special types of patients than other doctors and were distributed quite uniformly in all academic strata. Psychiatrists tended to be underrepresented in the top academic rank of their classes but tended to have high MCAT scores. They often cited special patient interests as an influence in selecting a field of practice, and more often than all doctors reported that they were born in a large city. While these differences are not as striking as those which distinguish the general practitioner from the teacher or researcher or from all specialists, there were, evidently, many patterns of influence upon the choices of students and trainees when they planned their training and their careers.

## DISCUSSION AND CONCLUSION

These findings illustrate, not surprisingly, that critical career decisions about the physician's field of practice, the length and quality of his training—and, by implication from other studies, the level of his competence—are influenced by multiple factors. Many are present before medical education begins, in backgrounds of students; others operate during undergraduate medical education and are functions of the school and the medical education process.

One of the surprising findings is the number and variety of differences between students in public and in private medical schools in our sample. We have examined these differences closely to see whether they represented an influence of medical school "environment" on career choices. It became clear that these differences are heavily influenced by the strikingly different proportions of future general practitioners (with the unique characteristics just cited) in public and private schools; future general practitioners comprise one of every three public school students in our sample, while the figure for private schools ranges from one in seven (in 1950) to one in twelve (in 1954); conversely, of course, the private schools had much greater representation than the public schools among future specialists. Indeed, the public school (in our sample) is increasingly the source of general practitioners, and the absolute increase in general practitioners from the 1950 to 1954 total class is entirely due to the public school contribution. If one adds to general practitioners the number who become internists—to create a "family doctor" category—then 57 percent of public school graduates fit this classification, as opposed to only 31 percent of the private school graduates. It is of further and related interest that teachers and researchers come twice as often, proportionately, from private schools.

Many of the apparent differences, then, between public and private schools may reflect this differential presence of future general practitioners. For example, private school graduates are much more likely than public school graduates to report the influence of intellectual interests on their career and training choices, while public school graduates—like the general practitioners as a group—are more likely to report the influence of interest in patients and of finances, less likely to receive support from parents, more likely to have high earnings while in medical school, and more likely to be married before entering medical school.

The same general practitioner factor seems to influence differences between public and private schools regarding internship and residency training. Some 90 percent of public school graduates obtained a rotating internship, compared with only 53–54 percent of private school graduates—but within the private school group, although the proportion of general practitioners was much lower, over 90 percent of these future general practitioners obtained a rotating internship. A much higher proportion of public than private school graduates planned an internship only, and a higher proportion terminated their training with internship; private school graduates, on the other hand, were more likely than public school graduates to obtain major teaching hospital internships, less likely to have no residency, more likely to have two years or more of residency training, more likely to have residencies in major teaching hospitals, and more likely to obtain specialty certification. These differences between public and private schools are, in fact, due almost entirely to the much greater proportion of future general practitioners in the public schools; when general practitioners are eliminated from consideration, one finds that there are no differences between

## DISCUSSION AND CONCLUSION

public and private schools with regard to the training of specialists or to plans for obtaining internships, partial residency, or specialty certification. Thus, for the future specialist, there seems little effect that can be attributed to a public versus a private medical school education.

Other seeming differences in the overall ecology of public and private schools also relate to the general practitioner effect—for example, the tendency for private school undergraduates to receive more encouragement from all sources, particularly from clinical chiefs, or the tendency of public school undergraduates to report more self-support as undergraduates.

There are, however, some differences between public and private schools within the category of future general practice; it is possibly a somewhat different matter, in our sample, to be an undergraduate bound for general practice (one in three) in a public school than in a private school (one in seven to one in twelve). Thus, two thirds of the general practice graduates of public schools terminated their training with internship, while only one third of the general practice graduates of private schools did so. Again, of all graduates who took a rotating internship, private school graduates were more likely—and public school graduates less likely—to go on to residency training. This may represent a public-private differential effective even after the common filter of a rotating internship, or it may relate simply to the varying proportions of general practitioners in public schools and private schools among those with rotating internships. Among all those who took straight internships, for example, there was no difference between public and private schools in the proportion going on to a residency.

The retrospective and evaluative views of public school graduates, as opposed to private school graduates, also probably reflect the greater proportion of general practitioners in the public school classes. Thus, the public school graduates in general (like general practitioners in general) were more likely to feel that their undergraduate medical education had failed them in some respect. Among general practitioners alone, two thirds of the public school graduates were dissatisfied, compared with only one half of the private school graduates.

We are reluctant to conclude, however, that differences between public and private schools are due exclusively to the varying presence of future general practitioners. The striking difference between public and private schools in output of general practitioners is in itself an important subject for further study. Its causes should be considered: the possibility that substantially different groups of applicants are drawn to the two kinds of schools, and the possibility that different (but as yet not specifically identified) selection processes are at work. It is important, furthermore, to know whether these differences in output persist over time, as well as to know more about the causes of more specific variations. Why is it, for example, that there are few differences in the training of specialist graduates of public and private schools while general practitioner graduates of private medical schools are likelier to obtain longer or "better" training than their counterparts in public schools? Farnsworth, Frothingham, and Wedge have emphasized that, at their most extreme, students can be characterized as "pragmatic" or "ideistic" and that educational results are best when these antipodal groups are placed in appropriate educational programs.* There is ample

---

* D. Farnsworth, D. H. Funkenstein, and B. Wedge, A Study of the Social and Emotional Adjustment of Early Admission Students, prepared for the Fund for the Advancement of Education, February 1956, as quoted in D. H. Funkenstein, "Possible Contributions of Psychological Testing of the Nonintellectual Characteristics of Applicants to Medical School," *Journal of Medical Education*, 32. 2:88–112 (October 1957).

## DISCUSSION AND CONCLUSION 223

evidence from our data that students destined for general practice have many compelling reasons for being pragmatically oriented. It is quite possible that the differences between general practitioner graduates of public and private schools may represent different degrees of selection and hence different degrees of pragmatism even within the general practitioner group. Our results, which are based upon a sample of only twelve schools, but are of high statistical significance, did not go as deeply into these major issues of the ecology of medical education. These questions will repay more intensive study.

The characteristics and social backgrounds of students and the students' experiences in medical school are insufficient in themselves, however, as a basis for the interpretation of our findings. There is a third major factor which we have referred to as the postgraduate training system. It is a matter of common knowledge within this system—among students, teachers, clinicians, internship and residency selection boards, and so forth—that there are a number of well-defined "tracks" that begin in undergraduate medical education and continue for some years thereafter. Students with higher class rank tend more to seek straight internships in major teaching hospitals, to be encouraged and recommended for these posts, and to be sought after by hospital selection boards. The appointment to such an internship tends to open a series of doors along a defined corridor of major teaching hospital residency, longer residency training, and specialty certification; the future teacher or researcher is the purest case. Conversely, students in the lowest class ranks tend to receive less encouragement and fewer recommendations, to seek rotating internships in nonteaching hospitals, and to be chosen for these posts; such a choice tends to close the doors to subsequent major teaching hospital training, to longer residencies, and to specialty certification, while leaving doors open along another corridor of shorter training in nonteaching institutions. Indeed, our data show that the character of the internship obtained was in fact predictive; different internships were associated with very different probabilities of both the length and the quality of further training. Thus, major teaching hospital internships were associated with greater probabilities of residency training; rotating internships in nonteaching hospitals were associated with greater probabilities that training would terminate without residency, that residency training—if obtained—would tend to be shorter, and that it would take place in hospitals other than major teaching institutions. The general practitioner is the purest case here.

It is this "system" that interacts with social, personal, and family background factors and with the medical education system that treats and encourages students differentially in the undergraduate medical years. It is the end products of this system —without much reference to the interaction of postgraduate training with social, personal, and undergraduate medical education factors—that have been examined in many of the studies of training and clinical competence.

Our data do not, of course, "prove" the existence of this system. For example, we have no information on unsuccessful applicants to the medical schools in our sample, nor on internships and residencies sought but not obtained by our sample of physicians, nor on the powerful (indeed, perhaps determining) role of hospital selection committees in the "choice" of training by medical students. Furthermore, our information is retrospective; the events reported to us, and (in particular) the reasons now cited for them, may not be the only ones, or the most powerful ones, actually operative at the time. Nevertheless, our data do support the existence of this postgraduate training

## DISCUSSION AND CONCLUSION 225

system in interaction with the social system that produces candidates for different medical schools and the medical education system that treats and encourages different groups of students differentially in their undergraduate medical years.

Thus, it is clear in our sample that where intellectual interests are cited as powerful, the training pathway is likely to be toward a straight internship in a major teaching hospital; where financial and social factors are cited as powerful, the training pathway is likely to involve rotating internships in nonteaching hospitals. These choices have both antecedent and subsequent associations. On the one hand, intellectual interests are associated with higher class rank, and financial factors with lower class rank. On the other hand—that is, prospectively—it is clear that a straight internship in a major teaching hospital is likely to lead to a residency, and a longer residency; a rotating internship in a major teaching hospital is likely to lead to residency, but of shorter average duration; while a rotating internship in a nonteaching hospital is likely to lead to the least residency, the least future association with a major teaching hospital, or no residency at all. These are the pathways that connect the pattern of a more highly educated father, younger age, and less financial pressure as an undergraduate (the social system); the pattern of high intellectual interest, high class rank, and frequent encouragement and support (the medical education system); and the association of each of these variables with the major teaching hospital internship, the longer residency, or the specialty certification (the postgraduate training system).

These associations abound in our data; for example, the findings that greater self-support is associated with greater frequency of rotating internship, while less self-support is associated with greater frequency of straight internship. The converse is true of parental support; its lack appears to be associated not only with greater frequency of rotating internship, but also with greater frequency of no residency, and its presence is associated with greater frequency of straight internship with residency and with greater frequency of long residency training. Early marriage, particularly marriage before entering medical school, has similar strong associations along the pathway whose way stations are frequently increased age, large debts, rotating internships, no residency, and the other factors which limit training.

Again, such associations or clusters of associations do not, of course, establish linear cause-and-effect relationships; this is why we must speak, however imprecisely at present, of the "interactions" or, as in the text, of "associations" of social, medical educational, and postgraduate training factors.

The timing of decisions about training may be particularly important in viewing these pathways and in deciding—if one so desires—where to intervene in an attempt to change them. Overall, for example, 10 percent of our physicians decided on their total amount of training while still in medical school, about two thirds while in medical school or during internship, and the remainder while in residency training. But of those with no residency, 50 percent made their final decision about total training during the internship that terminated their training. We know that those with rotating internships—particularly in nonteaching hospitals—are the likeliest to obtain no residency; this suggests an obvious point and time of intervention in an attempt to encourage further training. This is only one such point, however, and it seems likely that there will have to be others that occur much earlier. It is noteworthy, for example, that increased encouragement by parents and spouse, increased encouragement from clinical chiefs, increased parental support, and fewer finan

## DISCUSSION AND CONCLUSION 227

cial problems all are associated with greater frequency of straight internship and longer residency, and that these choices are also associated with early decision—while still in medical school—as to the total amount of training desired. In other words, a higher yield of straight internships and longer residency training—if either or both of these are desired—might be obtained by providing much more encouragement and more financial support in the early undergraduate years.

Indeed, the graduates of these various pathways, in our sample, seem to have retrospective views of their training that are quite consistent with an argument for attempts to intervene. Those with training in major teaching hospitals, and those with the longest residency, now express the least dissatisfaction with their medical education, while those with no residency now express the highest frequency of dissatisfaction. But perhaps (once again) intervention should be early: in retrospect, over 80 percent of the respondents were, overall, satisfied with their internships and residencies, but much less frequently satisfied with their undergraduate training.

Clearly, different factors are important at different points in time throughout the training cycle. Thus, in undergraduate years those with low class rank (who have a higher probability of ending with no residency) probably felt neglected since they reported less encouragement by the faculty; later, those who curtailed their hospital training stated most frequently that they did so for economic reasons.

In summary, what our data suggest—in considerable detail—is that varying groups of students, who differ in social and personal backgrounds, age, financial resources, marital status, and, to some extent but not greatly, in ability, obtain entry to medical school; that one fairly well-defined group of students tends to do poorly in school and another to do well; that the former receive less encouragement and support, the latter much more; and that those who have done less well are much more likely to enter a much shorter postgraduate training period, unassociated with the teaching hospitals, while those who have done better get the best and the longest training. Subsequently, shorter training in nonteaching hospitals is found to be associated with lower clinical competence, longer training in teaching hospitals with higher clinical competence.

By the triple measures, then, of measured clinical competence, satisfaction during undergraduate education, and satisfaction after training is completed, there is a high road and a low road in medical education. One may properly ask: Is this good for medical education? And, even more pertinently, is this good for society? If we conclude (as we must) that this situation is not best for society, what then can we do about it?

The first possibility is to do nothing and accept the fact that there are now, and in the future will be, both well trained and poorly trained physicians and that some will be less competent than they could be. Society has given ample evidence that it is interested in obtaining good medical care and that it prizes competence in its physicians. The high proportion of the American gross national product spent for medical care and the generous support of medical education and of medical research by both government and voluntary agencies all attest to the country's interest in good medical care and health. The recent history of medicine in the United States is concerned mainly with efforts to improve the quality of medical care through the improvement of medical education, improvements in hospitals, assuring the availability of medical care through orderly prepayment mech-

## DISCUSSION AND CONCLUSION

anisms, and the like. All indications point to the probability that the American public will support action that gives promise of improving medical care. Doing nothing may be impossible as well as short-sighted.

We could, of course, eliminate the students who take the low road through medical education by eliminating the medical school applicants who are married, who are older than their classmates, or who have limited financial resources, and later by eliminating the medical students who rank in the lower part of their class. This type of discrimination would eliminate many students whose training reaches an early dead end, but it would also eliminate some with these same limitations who prepare themselves long and well for practice. There are certainly better ways of meeting the problem than by denying opportunities to the students who have had to struggle for an education—especially at a time when medical education is being expanded to meet the needs of a growing population.

Some of the possible approaches are simple. We can help students understand the importance of training, the effects of different training choices upon their subsequent careers and clinical performance. Counseling and encouraging students to plan their training with a view to achieving clinical competence may be helpful, but the effect is likely to be marginal because students are confronted with realities that may be incompatible with their ideal choices.

It has been suggested that medical schools should assume responsibility for all medical training (specifically for nonteaching internships and residencies) with the object of improving these educational programs. Recently, the Millis Commission has recommended that "programs of graduate medical education be approved by the residency review committees only if they cover the entire span from the first year of graduate medical education through completion of the residency."(21) This and the accompanying recommendations that institutional responsibilities be substituted for service or individual responsibility as a prerequisite for accreditation of training program, if fulfilled, would ensure a higher standard for many of the internships with which general practitioners now conclude their training. A fully planned and complete training program would be a most important improvement. The strength of this proposal is emphasized by the experience of the general practitioners who received the least and poorest training and, more often than their classmates, reported that they terminated their training because of its poor quality. On the other hand, improvements in training programs are important in themselves, but they do not suggest a solution to the problems faced by the young intern with an empty pocketbook and family responsibilities.

Medical schools have slowly—almost at a glacial pace—extended their responsibilities for students over the years, often in reacting to social needs. For example, the practice of dropping the academically weaker students has largely been eliminated, in part because of better selections, but also as a reaction to the increasing need for physicians for a growing population. The expansion of major teaching hospital internships and residencies, for reasons often unrelated to training needs, has made available more of these desirable positions. Although we have no systematic information, it appears that more schools are actively helping students to plan their training programs, though even this minimum is absent in some schools. There is also discussion among medical educators about extending medical school responsibilities for internship, residency, and specialist certification, but this

## DISCUSSION AND CONCLUSION 231

falls short of meeting the problem of physicians who obtain training outside teaching hospitals. Many of the restrictions upon training cannot be solved by medical schools alone, of course. We do not know to what extent the relationship of marriage, greater age, and self-support during medical school or lack of parental support—all of which are associated with foreshortened training—may be expressions of economic constraints. The financial problems, in any case, are the only ones that have an easily identifiable solution—money.

Medical students, whose overall training period is longer than any other graduate student group, have received little financial aid in the past and still receive less than graduate students in economics, biology, or physics—who expect substantial government or other fellowships for completing Ph.D. programs almost as a matter of course. The neglect of medical students, furthermore, stands in marked contrast to the government aid to physicians who enter training programs in undermanned fields such as psychiatry or public health. This restricted aid is offered at too late a stage to meet the problems of some medical school graduates, and its categorical approach has assured the neglect of a large group whose need for help is greatest.

It is perfectly clear that financial problems are involved at every stage of training including the internship and residency. The very low pay given to interns and to residents has been justified because of the learning benefits that accrue to the trainees. Society pays for this policy by accepting the fact that many doctors are poorly trained and that among this group most will be less competent than they could be and many will be less competent than is desirable. If interns and residents were to be paid sufficiently well so that they would be encouraged to pursue training until they had obtained maximum benefit, the direct cost to hospitals and to patients would be increased. These costs would be balanced by generally better patient care. The costs of less competent care are widely scattered and well hidden, but they are nonetheless very large—and they are always paid. We are, indeed, now being penny-wise and pound-foolish.*

Our data again and again indicate that the financial barrier is an important one and strongly suggests that its removal would eliminate a major deterrent to longer training within the multiply disadvantaged group who take the low road in training. Even if adequate pay would not induce all physicians to obtain adequate training, this should not argue against its use to accomplish a desirable objective. No single remedy will solve all problems and it should not be rejected because it does not.

Keppel has emphasized that it is characteristic of all education that it opens opportunities to the very able and neglects the least able. (17) The consequences of this educational practice will be concentrated upon the individual, but they also, as in medicine, have their social costs. The group of doctors in our sample who selected careers in teaching and research exemplify this process well. This group with high ability seemed to have few family or social problems that limited their training, were more frequently recipients of scholarships, and were often encouraged by the faculty in planning their careers. The general practitioners, whom we have repeatedly characterized as antipodal to the

---

\* The lack of wisdom in our present policy appears strongly when we examine society's interest in internship and residency training. While the physician in training benefits greatly from this training, he is also, for the first time, contributing in an important and substantial way to society. If the internship and the residency were to be abolished, the cost to society of replacing the large volume of lost patient services would add enormously to the total medical care bill. This is true whether we consider the circumscribed, but necessary, responsibilities of the new intern or the highly technical and sophisticated services rendered by a chief resident in surgery.

## DISCUSSION AND CONCLUSION 233

teaching and research group, were encumbered by many social and family problems and probably were most in need of attention, but they seem to have received much less than all other students. While it is perhaps natural to concentrate attention upon the very able, it is more important from the point of view of the end results that more attention be given to the least able students whose needs are greatest.

There are many signs that medical schools are becoming increasingly willing to deal with the fact that students learn and achieve competence at different rates. This interest is usually expressed in programs which allow the very able to accelerate their education; its full benefit will be realized only if the needs of the slower students receive their quota of attention. There is a distressing tendency at present to allow the borderline student, who is only the most extreme example, to graduate and to intern in a weak internship program because this is the only one open to him. It is, of course, precisely this student who needs good and prolonged training. Clinical medicine is not so complicated that it cannot be learned by the academically weaker members, if they were given more time in good internships and residencies. Although faculties often concern themselves with the "fundamentals" of medical education, this one—the relation between student ability and time devoted to learning—almost never receives attention.

The Millis Commission was concerned mainly with "comprehensive and continuing health care" for which they prescribed a new type of specialist, the primary physician. In commenting upon the type of care given by such a doctor, the report stated, "There are not enough such men and there is not enough of the service which they offer—as most patients, physicians and legislators agree." If action is taken to meet this shortage, it will be necessary to admit more and presumably academically weaker students to medical schools. Then the problem of how to obtain competent physicians from less promising recruits will have to be faced.

The very skewed nature of the selection of medical students from the population raises another problem for medical schools. Medical educators have set great store by the choices which they can make in selecting their student bodies in planning for an improved educational result. This is, of course, a very fundamental element in maintaining the quality of practice, but it is, at the same time, a very uncertain one with respect to the future. When American universities were founded, their function was mainly to prepare men for the ministry in a religious society. The early addition of law and medicine to university programs has been followed by increasingly rapid diversification of educational programs in every institution. The rapid proliferation of careers opened up by broadened university educational programs make it very unlikely that the choices which medical schools can make in selecting students will in the long run "improve" radically as long as the selection from the population is as highly skewed as it is at present. If there is to be any increase of choices enjoyed by educational institutions, including medical schools, the small number of students selected from blue collar and other occupational groups with low average income and generally limited educational family backgrounds will have to be increased. It is difficult to believe that the small number of medical students selected from the low average income families exhausts the students of high ability which this large segment of the population contains. Negroes, who comprise 11 percent of the United States population but only 2 percent of its physicians, represent an especially dramatic example of a neglected reservoir of talent. It is far from our minds to propose that medical schools should

DISCUSSION AND CONCLUSION 235

take direct responsibility for improving the quality of primary and grammar school education, or for accomplishing the broad social changes necessary to increase both opportunity and educational motivation for low-income populations, but medical educators must share with all other educators a deep concern and a willingness to commit themselves, when opportunities present, to remedy these shortcomings of our society.

Though medical educational change is urgently needed, no change—however massive—in the undergraduate or postgraduate medical training systems alone can achieve our goals of an adequate supply of well-trained, maximally competent physicians. This goal is extremely important to the social order. But the problems begin in this same sector—the social order. It is American society as a whole—the public, the legislators, and not just the medical schools—that must decide whether to extend the opportunity for a medical career to larger and lower-income populations and to pay the necessary costs, just as it is this larger society that will, alternatively, pay the costs of an inadequate physician supply or of low clinical competence.

But this social and educational goal—an adequate supply of well-trained, maximally competent physicians—is only one component of a still larger and overriding social goal: adequate, high-quality health services for everyone in the society. Clearly, this is not to be achieved merely by the production of physicians. Conversely, the larger social goal—the health care system—has enormous impact on the training of competent doctors. One need only realize, for example, how much social definition is built into the idea of our "adequate" supply of physicians; we are currently experiencing a major social redefinition of "adequate" in the commitments made by Medicare and Title 19 legislation alone.

This larger problem, and its influence on the training of physicians, has both quantitative and qualitative dimensions. Some of the quantitative implications have already been discussed: we will need more physicians, more medical schools, and therefore more recruits to medical education, and we will have to make special efforts to see that the "deprived" candidate and the "deprived" medical student—in our data, the future general practitioner—has real access to training of greater length and higher quality.*

The qualitative dimension refers to the organization and delivery of medical care, the funding of care, the training and use of para-professionals, the relationships between teaching hospitals and community hospitals—in short, the setting in which the future physician will work, the tasks he will undertake (or delegate to others), and the way in which he will work. The larger social issue of our adequate health care system involves far more than physicians alone, their technical quality or their competence. Indeed, the setting may in some measure influence how "competence" is to be defined. It is easy to say physicians must have good training—but training for what?

In this sense, there is a curiously narrow cast to much of the current, intense discussion of the disappearance of the general practitioner, the need for a "primary physician" with this or that training, or the merits of single-physician versus multiple-physician or multiple-specialty models of care. Frequent reference is made to the goal of "comprehensive care"; yet even when we

---

* It is probable that everything we have said about the hospital training of the student who now becomes a general practitioner holds true for the training of the foreign-born, foreign-trained physicians who are now, and will be for some time to come, an important component of our physician manpower. Evidence from many other studies indicates that most of them receive "dead-end training" in nonteaching hospitals; if we cannot, as a society, afford inferior postgraduate training for any of our own doctors, then we cannot afford it—and should not tolerate it—for foreign-trained physicians either.

## DISCUSSION AND CONCLUSION 237

talk about it we fail, far too often, to recognize it as a comprehensive problem—involving not merely physicians (whether generalist or specialist) but also nurses, social workers, technicians, numerous para-professionals, and many others (the so-called subprofessionals emerging as members of health teams) whose roles are yet to be defined clearly; and involving not merely health manpower but the financing and organization of their work. It is in this sense, we feel, that some of the debate over the merits of "primary physician" versus specialist, without reference to the larger or more comprehensive picture, resembles the discussions of angels and heads of pins. Good quality of training and performance, as we now define them for physicians, cannot and must not be neglected—but these may not be the only dimensions of quality important for the future. An increasing proportion of women are admitted to medical school; their full contribution to medicine will require adaptations that do not impose drastic choices, as is now so common, between residency training or a practice on the one hand and a family on the other. To cite but one more example, too few medical schools now give their undergraduates any coherent or intensive experience in partnership with such other professionals as visiting nurse or social worker. Our argument here is not for one or another particular new dimension of undergraduate or postgraduate training, but rather for recognition of the fact that what is considered important in physicians' training must be under continual review in dimensions beyond technical content.

Indeed, despite all the intensity of discussion and effort devoted to curriculum revision in many medical schools, our study may be interpreted as suggesting a powerful, entrenched conservatism in medical education. No matter how fondly medical schools may regard themselves as pioneers and innovators, the facts of the present study suggest that (in interaction with the social system and the postgraduate training system) they are dedicated to the status quo ante—producing either relatively poorly trained physicians for solo general practice or superbly trained physicians equipped for teaching and research in academic medical centers. These polar-paired models, existing in minimal relationship to each other, may represent yesterday's patterns of medical practice, but not tomorrow's. Few of the recent important innovations in medical care—for example, multiple varieties of group practice, experimental comprehensive neighborhood health centers, the increasing use of paramedical personnel and subprofessionals, the applications of computer and engineering technologies—are reflected as yet in the undergraduate curriculum. Medical schools cannot and should not be the sole arbiters of tomorrow's patterns of practice, but it seems to us they have a responsibility, at the least, for the training of students in ways that will permit much greater flexibility of subsequent education and participation in the medical care system. There is no mirror for the future—but we need not, therefore, merely reflect the past.

It is, we recognize clearly, much easier to raise such questions than to provide answers—but if the function of research is, in part, to raise new questions, we hope some of these will be among the questions considered in response to the present study.

**References**

**Index**

# References

1. Stuart Adams, "Trends in Occupational Origins of Physicians," *American Journal of Sociology*, 62:360–368 (January 1957).
2. Howard Becker, et al., *Boys in White* (Chicago, Illinois: University of Chicago Press, 1961).
3. J. H. F. Brotherston, F. M. Martin, and F. A. Boddy, Interim Report of the Medical Student Inquiry, Association for the Study of Medical Education, January 1963, mimeographed.
4. R. C. Buxbaum, to be published.
5. Joseph Ceithaml, "The Financial State of the American Medical Student," *Journal of Medical Education*, 40:498–499 (June 1965).
6. K. F. Clute, *The General Practitioner: A Study of Medical Education and Practice in Ontario and Nova Scotia* (Toronto: University of Toronto Press, 1963).
7. W. G. Cochran, *Sampling Techniques* (2nd ed., New York: John Wiley and Sons, 1963), pp. 64–65.
8. James Coleman, Elihu Katz, and Herbert Menzel, "The Diffusion of an Innovation among Physicians," *Sociometry*, 20:255 (December 1957).
9. J. J. Conger and R. H. Fitz, "Prediction of Success in Medical School," *Journal of Medical Education*, 38:943–948 (November 1963).
10. F. G. Dickenson, *Distribution of Medical School Alumni in the U.S. as of April 1950* (Chicago, Illinois: American Medical Association, 1955).
11. Helen H. Gee and Robert J. Glazer, eds., *The Ecology of the Medical Student* (Evanston, Illinois: Association of American Medical Colleges, 1958).
12. H. C. Gough, W. B. Hall, and R. E. Harris, "Admissions Procedures as Forecasters of Performance in Medical Training," *Journal of Medical Education*, 38:983–998 (December 1963).
13. Kenneth R. Hammond, et al., *Teaching Comprehensive Medical Care* (Cambridge, Massachusetts: Harvard University Press, 1959).
14. V. H. Jensen and M. H. Clark, "Married and Unmarried College Students: Achievement, Ability, and Personality," *Personnel and Guidance Journal*, 37:123–125 (October 1958).
15. D. G. Johnson, "An 'Actuarial' Approach to Medical Student Selection," *Journal of Medical Education*, 35:158–163 (February 1960).

16. D. G. Johnson, "A Multifactor Method of Evaluating Medical School Applicants," *Journal of Medical Education*, 37:656–665 (July 1962).
17. Francis Keppel, *The Necessary Revolution in American Education* (New York, New York: Harper and Row, 1966).
18. A. J. Kubany, "Use of Sociometric Peer Nominations in Medical Education Research," *Journal of Applied Psychology*, 41:389–394 (June 1957).
19. Robert Merton, et al., *The Student Physician* (Cambridge, Massachusetts: Harvard University Press, 1957).
20. R. L. Millikin and J. A. Samensink, "Marital Status and Academic Success: A Reconsideration," *Marriage and Family Living*, 23:226–227 (August 1961).
21. John S. Millis, et al., *The Graduate Education of Physicians—The Report of the Citizens Commission on Graduate Medical Education* (Chicago, Illinois: American Medical Association, 1966).
22. M. A. Morehead, "Quality of Medical Care Provided by Family Physicians as Related to Their Education, Training and Methods of Practice," Health Insurance Plan of New York, mimeographed.
23. O. L. Peterson, L. P. Andrews, R. S. Spain, and B. G. Greenberg, "An Analytical Study of North Carolina General Practice," *Journal of Medical Education*, 31.2:1–165 (December 1956).
24. O. L. Peterson, F. J. Lyden, H. J. Geiger, and T. Colton, "Appraisal of Medical Students' Abilities as Related to Training and Careers after Graduation," *New England Journal of Medicine*, 269:1174–1182 (November 1963).
25. S. Riemer, "Married Veterans Are Good Students," *Marriage and Family Living*, 9:11–12 (February 1947).
26. C. F. Schumacher, "A Factor-Analytic Study of Various Criteria of Medical Students' Accomplishments," *Journal of Medical Education*, 39:192–196 (February 1964).
27. A. E. Schwartzman, R. C. A. Hunter, and J. G. Lohrenz, "Factors Related to Student Withdrawals from Medical Schools," *Journal of Medical Education*, 37:1114–1120 (October 1962).
28. L. Soutter, "Student Finances," *Journal of Medical Education*, 33:380–388 (April 1958).
29. H. G. Weiskotten, et al., "Trends in Medical Practice—An Analysis of the Distribution and Characteristics of Medical College Graduates," *Journal of Medical Education*, 35:1071–1121 (December 1960).

# Index

Academic measures, 89–95, 118–125
Age, 26–29, 63–66, 138–145

Birthplace, 61–63, 137–138

Certification, Specialty Board, 23, 24, 25, 98–99, 185
Class esteem, 81, 170–174
Class rank: and field of practice, 92–95; and influences on field of practice decisions, 112–114; training variables, 122–125; and father's education, 126; and mother's education, 128; and birthplace, 137–138; and age, 139, 141; and sources of support, 145, 146, 153; and debt at graduation, 158; and marital status, 164, 168; and class esteem, 171; and friendships, 173–174; and encouragement to continue training beyond internship, 181, 183; and certification, 185; and satisfaction with training, 189, 196–197, 198; of general practitioners, 216

Data analysis, 12–14
Debt at graduation, 72–75, 158–163
Deprivations, 75–76, 163–164

Earnings while in medical school, 68, 69, 71–72, 152–158
Economic circumstances, 66–76, 163–164, 200–202, 204
Encouragement to continue training beyond internship, 99, 102–103, 176–185

Family background, 54–60, 73–75, 125–137, 214; father's education, 54–55, 125–128, 214; and field of practice, 55, 58–59; father's occupation, 57–58, 73, 75, 132–137, 214; father's age, 60; and MCAT, 126–128; and class rank, 126–128; and training, 126–128, 130, 131, 132–138; mother's education, 128, 130; father's ethnic origin, 130–131, 132; mother's ethnic origin, 131–132
Family composition, 60–61
Family doctors, 21, 22
Field of practice: numbers and percents, 19–22; certification, 24–26, 99; and age, 27, 29, 64, 66; and type of practice, 31, 33–34, 36; and present location of practice, 39; and practice income, 42–44; and value orientation, 46; and marital status, 46, 77, 79; influences on field of practice decisions, 51–54, 104–105, 110, 111, 112; and father's education, 55; and father's occupation, 58–59; and father's ethnic origin, 59; and birthplace, 61, 63; and sources of support, 68, 69, 72, 73, 75; and friendships, 81; and hospital training, 81–89; and MCAT, 91–92; and class rank, 92–95; and time of decision about amount of training, 96; and encouragement to continue training beyond internship, 102–103; and satisfaction with training, 187, 195, 197–198; training choices in retrospect, 205, 206, 208–211; general practitioners, 215–217; teachers and researchers, 217–218
Friendships and career choices, 80–81, 172–175

General practitioners: numbers and percents, 19–22; amount of training planned, 24–25, 99; age, 27, 29, 64, 66, 215; type of practice, 31, 33, 34, 217; present location of practice, 39; practice income, 42, 217; value orientation, 46; marital status, 46, 79, 215; influences on field of practice decisions, 51–53, 105, 216; father's education, 55, 125–128, 215;

father's occupation, 58–59, 132–137, 215; father's ethnic origin, 59, 130–131, 132; father's age, 60; family composition, 61; birthplace, 61, 63, 216; sources of support, 68–69, 72, 73, 216; earnings while in medical school, 72, 152; debt at graduation, 73; hospital training, 83–84, 86, 88–89, 216–217; MCAT, 91–92, 216; class rank, 94, 216; time of decisions about amount of training, 96; encouragement to continue training beyond internship, 102–103, 216; satisfaction with training, 187, 195, 197–198; reasons for curtailment of training, 201–202; training choices in retrospect, 209, 211

Hospital appointments, 41

Income from practice, 41–45
Influences on field of practice decisions, 44–45, 104–114
Interaction of social, medical education, and postgraduate training systems, 213–228
Internists: numbers and percents, 21; age, 27, 29; type of practice, 34; practice income, 42; value orientation, 46; marital status, 46, 79; influences on field of practice decisions, 53, 105; father's ethnic origin, 59; sources of support, 68–69; MCAT, 92; class rank, 94; time of decisions about amount of training, 96; encouragement to continue training beyond internship, 103; training choices in retrospect, 209, 211

Marital status, 46, 77–80, 164–169, 214
MCAT: and field of practice, 89–92; and influences on field of practice decisions, 114; and training variables, 118–122; and father's education, 126; and mother's education, 128; and birthplace, 137; and age, 139; and sources of support, 145, 146, 153; and earnings while in medical school, 153; and debt at graduation, 158; and marital status, 164–165, 168; and class esteem, 171; and encouragement to continue training beyond internship, 183; and certification, 185; and satisfaction with training, 187–189, 196, 198; for general practitioners, 216–218
Medical education, suggestions for improvement, 228–233

Obstetricians and gynecologists, 54, 84, 105

Pediatricians, 54, 105
Practice, 29–39
Psychiatrists, 46, 63, 81

Questionnaire, 10–12

Respondents: diversity, 1, 212–214; backgrounds, 1, 212–213, 214, 215–216

Sample, 6–10
Satisfaction with training, 186–197
Schools, differences between public and private, 215–223
Significance, tests of, 14–16, 20
Support: sources of, 66–75, 145–163; and MCAT, 145, 146, 153; and class rank, 145, 146, 153; and training, 148–152, 153–163
Surgeons: numbers and percents, 21, 22; age, 27, 29; type of practice, 36; practice income, 42, 44; value orientation, 46; influences on field of practice decisions, 53; family composition, 61; sources of support, 68–69; marital status, 79; class rank, 94; time of decisions about amount of training, 96; encouragement to continue training beyond internship, 103; training choices in retrospect, 205–206, 209, 211

Teachers and researchers: numbers and percents, 21–22; age, 27, 29, 64; value orientation, 46; influences on field of practice decisions, 53, 105; father's education, 55; father's occupation, 59; birthplace, 63; friendships, 81; class esteem, 81; training, 84, 86, 89; MCAT for, 92; class rank, 94–95; time of decision about amount of training, 96; encouragement to continue training beyond internship, 103

Terms defined, 16–18

Training: amount planned, 22–26, 96, 98–99; and field of practice, 81–89; decisions about, 95–103, 175–176; influences on field of practice decisions, 105, 107, 109–112; interrelationship of training variables, 114–118; MCAT and, 118–122; and family background, 126, 128, 130, 131, 132–137; and birthplace, 138; and age, 141–145; and sources of support, 145–158; and debt at graduation, 158–163; and marital status, 165–169; and class esteem, 171–172; and friendships, 174; certification, 185; satisfaction with, 189–191, 193, 195, 197–200; reasons for curtailment of, 200–204; choices in retrospect, 204–211

Value orientation, 45–46

Wives, views of, 169–170